Muscular Dystrophy and Other Neuromuscular Diseases: Psychosocial Issues

Muscular Dystrophy and Other Neuromuscular Diseases: Psychosocial Issues

Leon I. Charash, Robert E. Lovelace, Claire F. Leach,
Austin H. Kutscher, Rabbi Jacob Goldberg,
David Price Roye, Jr.
Editors

Jill C. Crabtree
Editor for the Foundation of Thanatology

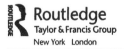

Routledge
Taylor & Francis Group
New York   London

Routledge is an imprint of the
Taylor & Francis Group, an informa business

Muscular Dystrophy and Other Neuromuscular Diseases: Psychosocial Issues has also been published as *Loss, Grief & Care*, Volume 4, Numbers 3/4 1990.

Reprinted 2009 by Routledge

Library of Congress Cataloging-in-Publication Data

Muscular dystrophy and other neuromuscular diseases : psychosocial issues / Leon I. Charash . . . [et al.], editors, Jill C. Crabtree, editor for the Foundation of Thanatology.
    p. cm.
    Also published as: Loss, grief & care, v.4, no. 3/4 1990
    ISBN 1-56024-077-6 (alk paper)
    1. Neuromuscular diseases — Psychological aspects. 2. Neuromuscular diseases — Social aspects. 3. Muscular dystrophy — Psychological aspects. 4. Muscular dystrophy — Social aspects. I. Charash, Leon I.
    [DNLM: 1. Muscular Dystrophy — psychology. 2. Neuromuscular Diseases — psychology. W1 L0853F v. 4 no. 3/4 / WE 550 M9856]
RC925.M83 1990
616.7'44 — dc20
DNLM/DLC
for Library of Congress

91-6992
CIP

Muscular Dystrophy and Other Neuromuscular Diseases: Psychosocial Issues

CONTENTS

ABOUT THE EDITORS

Leon I. Charash is Chairman of the Medical Advisory Committee of the Muscular Dystrophy Association, Incorporated. He is also Associate Professor of Pediatrics at Cornell University Medical Center in New York City.

Robert E. Lovelace, MD, FRCP, is Professor of Neurology at the College of Physicians and Surgeons, Columbia University in New York, New York, where he has worked for over twenty-seven years as a faculty member and a practicing neurologist. He is also Co-Director of the Muscular Dystrophy Clinic at Columbia-Presbyterian Medical Center in New York City.

Claire F. Leach is Clinical Social Worker in the Department of Neurology of the Nassau County Medical Center in East Meadow, New York.

Austin H. Kutscher, PhD, is President of The Foundation of Thanatology and Professor of Dentistry (in Psychiatry) at the College of Physicians and Surgeons of Columbia University in New York City. His clinical and teaching activities have focused on psychosocial aspects of life-threatening illness and bereavement; cancer diagnosis, therapy, and management; and pharmacotherapeutics.

Rabbi Jacob Goldberg is Director of the Commission on Pastoral Bereavement Counseling and also Assistant Professor for Bereavement Counseling at the Wurzweiler School of Social Work at Yeshiva University in New York City.

David Price Roye, Jr., MD, is Assistant Professor of Clinical Orthopedic Surgery in the Department of Orthopedic Surgery of the College of Physicians and Surgeons at Columbia University in New York City.

Muscular Dystrophy and Other Neuromuscular Diseases: Psychosocial Issues

Preface

Life has many challenges, and dealing with the difficulties imposed by a chronic disability is certainly a tremendous one. The news of the diagnosis of a severe medical problem often comes as a great shock to the patient as well as family members. Not only are there feelings of guilt, fear, blame, and stress, which exact a toll in family relationships, but the prospect of living with a chronic progressive physical disability may lead to a good deal of anxiety, doubts, and questions—which cry out for resolution.

Often efforts are made to seek opinion after opinion in the hope that someone will disprove the diagnosis and alleviate the fears and dread of a progressive illness. When such efforts fail to secure a less dire diagnosis, a sense of intense aloneness may engulf the entire family. But they are not alone. There are many concerned professionals who care deeply and are prepared to offer their support and professional guidance.

This text reports on the findings of professionals who, over the years, have developed strategies for maintaining the psychosocial well-being of youngsters and adults with chronic, progressive neuromuscular disorders, as well as that of family members. The Muscular Dystrophy Association is pleased to have been of assistance in the publication of this important book.

Ronald J. Schenkenberger

Ronald J. Schenkenberger is Director of Patient and Community Services, Muscular Dystrophy Association, New York, NY.

SECTION I:
PSYCHOSOCIAL ASPECTS
OF NEUROMUSCULAR DISORDERS

Impact of Illness on Lifestyle

Lisa B. Schwartz
Patricia A. Devine
Clyde B. Schechter
Adam N. Bender

The percentage of our population with chronic and terminal illness is on the rise, largely due to increasing numbers of elderly and advances in medical technology and chemotherapy (Forsyth, Delaney, and Gresham 1984; Wilson and Drury 1984). Cost containment is now a major issue in the health arena, causing a shift in treatment from long-term hospital stays

Lisa B. Schwartz, MD, is affiliated with the Department of Neurology; Patricia A. Devine, MD, is affiliated with the Neuromuscular Clinic; Clyde B. Schechter, MD, is Assistant Professor of Community Medicine; and Adam N. Bender, MD, is Associate Professor of Neurology and Director of the Neuromuscular Clinic and Laboratory, all at Mount Sinai Hospital and Medical Center, New York, NY 10029.

This work was submitted in partial fulfillment of the clerkship requirements in Community Medicine while Patricia Devine and Lisa Schwartz were third-year students at Mount Sinai School of Medicine.

The authors wish to thank Virginia Walther, CSW, for help with this investigation.

to ambulatory care. As a result, there is a need to reevaluate whether the psychosocial needs of the chronically and terminally ill are being met within this changing system.

The purpose of this study is to explore the similarities and differences between patients with myasthenia gravis (MG), a chronic disease, and amyotrophic lateral sclerosis (ALS), a terminal disease. Both are neuromuscular diseases characterized by muscle weakness, and both can lead to difficulty in talking and swallowing as well as to difficulty in breathing, life on a respirator, and death (Muscular Dystrophy Association 1984, 1986; Myasthenia Gravis Foundation 1985; Sivak, Gipson, and Hanson 1982; Charles 1985). The similarity of these two diseases led Mulder, Lambert and Eaton in 1959 to address the issue of confusion of the two diagnoses in their article "Myasthenic Syndrome in Patients with Amyotrophic Lateral Sclerosis." This internal consistency makes these two diseases ideal in studying the larger hypothesis since MG is treatable and ALS is not.

MG is an autoimmune disease caused by a reduction in the number of functioning acetylcholine receptors in the muscle endplate (Myasthenia Gravis Foundation 1985, 1986). This causes abnormal neuromuscular transmission and results in voluntary muscle fatigue, ptosis, and diplopia. It most commonly affects women of childbearing age and men in their fifth decade (Myasthenia Gravis Foundation 1985). The treatment of MG includes anticholinesterase agents, thymectomy, steroids and other immunosuppressive drugs, and plasmapheresis (Muscular Dystrophy Association 1986; Myasthenia Gravis Foundation 1986).

ALS is a disease cf unknown etiology in which the upper and lower motor neurons gradually disintegrate, resulting in progressive atrophy of the muscle cells they innervate (Muscular Dystrophy Association 1984). Muscular atrophy, paralysis, fasciculations, hyperreflexia, emotional incontinence, and relentless progression are characteristic (Myasthenia Gravis Foundation 1985; Udaka et al. 1984). It occurs more commonly in men (1.5 male:1.0 female) with the average age of onset 57 years old. Fifty percent of all ALS patients die within three years of onset (Janiszewski, Caroscio, and Wisham 1983).

METHODS

In order to evaluate the differences in the impact on lifestyle of a treatable diagnosis versus an untreatable one, a cross-sectional survey design was utilized. The study population was composed of 19 ALS and 19 MG patients from the respective clinics at Mount Sinai Medical Center, which is a national center for ALS and a regional center for MG. Twenty-two questionnaires were distributed to ALS patients and 20 to MG patients; 39 were completed for a response rate of 93%. Three ALS patients dropped out.

Almost all the instruments in this study have already been used and extensively pretested where their validity and reliability have been established (Wallston et al. 1976; Billings and Moos 1981; Brown, Rawlinson, and Hilles 1981; Schipper and Levitt 1985; Spitzer et al. 1981). The survey form contained a total of eight sections of fill-in, multiple choice and yes/no questions:

1. Demographics. This included date of birth, sex, race, marital status, education, occupation, income, and date of diagnosis.

2. Severity of Illness. The patient rated his concept of illness severity as compared to the physician's assessment. Swallowing and breathing difficulties were included because these are common manifestations of very advanced stages in both illnesses.

3. Coping Styles. This was adapted from the Billings and Moos (1981) coping response items. Included are three methods of coping and two foci of coping categories. Coping methods consisted of active cognitive (AC) coping (6 items), including attempts to manage one's appraisal of the stressfulness of the event; active behavioral (AB) coping (6 items), referring to overt behavioral attempts to deal directly with the problem and its effects; and avoidance coping (5 items), referring to attempts to avoid actively confronting the problem or to indirectly reduce emotional tension by eating or smoking more. Coping foci consisted of problem-focused (PF) coping (6 items), including attempts to modify or eliminate the sources of stress through one's own behavior; and emotion-focused (EF) coping (11 items), including behavioral or cognitive responses whose primary function is to manage the emotional consequences of stressors and to help maintain one's emotional equilibrium (Billings and Moos 1981).

4. Life Satisfaction, Perceived Health and Social Activity. Brown et al. (1981) proposed a life satisfaction model where they compared coronary artery disease with chronic obstructive pulmonary disease patients. Life satisfaction, perceived health, and social activity were each measured by a 9-Rung Cantril Ladder, which is an equal-interval, self-anchoring scale.

5. Multidimensional Health Locus of Control (MHLC). MHLC is an 18-item Likert-type instrument developed by Wallston et al. and based on Rotter's social learning theory (Wallston et al. 1976; Wallston and Wallston 1978). It consists of subscales reflecting three dimensions: whether the patients think (1) they have control over their health (internal LOC); (2) their health is determined by powerful others (external LOC); or (3) their health is a matter of luck (chance LOC). Items are scored on a six-point scale and answers are totaled as three separate scores (McFarlane et al. 1980).

6. *Psychosocial Well-Being*. This section explored social life, family relations, friendships, recreation, religious activities, and psychological well-being. Seven out of the 14 questions (4, 5, 10, 11, 12, 13 and 14) were adapted from the Functional Living Index for Cancer (FLIC) (Schipper and Levitt 1985) (see Table 1). FLIC is a 22-item survey that utilizes the Likert Scale. The polarities of the questions were alternated in FLIC. We modified this by arranging all negative polarities on the left side and positive polarities on the right side since Corney and Clare's (1985) pilot study on the Social Problem Questionnaire showed that alternating directions causes confusion. Questions 6, 7 and 8 were adapted from Ware, who emphasized the importance of social factors in conceptualizing disease impact (Ware 1984; Holahan and Moos 1981). Questions 2, 3 and 9 were innovative questions.

7. *Public and Body Image*. This section examined distorted body image and lack of privacy, two changes often found in chronic and terminal illness according to Purtilo (1976). It consisted of three yes/no questions: (1) Since the diagnosis, do you ever find yourself hesitating to look in the mirror? (2) When you go out in public, do you feel like people are staring at you? and (3) If yes, has this caused you to avoid public places? The last two questions compared type of diagnosis and public image.

8. *Quality of Life (QOL)*. QOL of the two groups was compared by using the "Q-L INDEX" developed by Spitzer et al. (1981). The Q-L INDEX consists of five distinct item groups including activity, daily living, health, support, and outlook. Each item is scored on a 0-2 point scale giving a total score of 0-10.

RESULTS

The mean age was greater for ALS (61.91) than for MG (53.59) whereas the standard deviation was greater for MG than for ALS patients (Table 2). This age difference was taken into account in the analysis by comparing age-specific scores of the 15 MG patients 40 years old or older with the ALS group for all lifestyle variables. A younger subgroup could not be compared since a younger age group did not exist for ALS. There were also some discrepancies in the distribution of perceived illness severity between the two groups (Table 3). There was a small subgroup that regarded their illness as mild, and they were equally represented in the two diseases. Ratios of moderate and advanced were reversed in the two

Table 1 PSYCHOSOCIAL WELL-BEING

Please circle the number that you feel best describes you on each of the scales below.

1. What was your initial reaction to your diagnosis?

   1   2   3   4   5   6   7

   rejection   acceptance

2. How long after you were told your diagnosis did you tell your family and friends?

   1   2   3   4   5   6   7

   long time   short time

3. Rate whether this has drawn you and your family closer together or further apart.

   1   2   3   4   5   6   7

   further   closer
   apart   together

4. Rate in your opinion how disruptive your disease has been to those closest to you.

   1   2   3   4   5   6   7

   totally   no
   disruptive   disruption

5. Rate how willing you are to see and spend time with your friends.

   1   2   3   4   5   6   7

   unwilling   very
                                         willing

6. Since your diagnosis, has the number of your friends changed?

   1   2   3   4   5   6   7

   decreased   increased
   a lot   a lot

7. Since your diagnosis, has the frequency of visits with friends and relatives changed?

   1   2   3   4   5   6   7

   decreased   increased
   a lot   a lot

TABLE 1 (continued)

8. Since your diagnosis, has the number of club and organizational memberships changed?

1	2	3	4	5	6	7
decreased a lot						increased a lot

9. Since your diagnosis, has the frequency of your attendance at religious services changed?

1	2	3	4	5	6	7
decreased a lot						increased a lot

10. Rate your ability to maintain your usual recreational or leisure activities.

1	2	3	4	5	6	7
unable						able

11. How much time do you spend thinking about your illness?

1	2	3	4	5	6	7
constantly						never

12. How well are you coping with everyday stress?

1	2	3	4	5	6	7
not well						very well

13. Rate how often you feel discouraged about your life.

1	2	3	4	5	6	7
always						never

14. Rate the degree to which you are frightened of the future.

1	2	3	4	5	6	7
constantly terrified						not afraid

TABLE 2 - AGE, SEX AND NUMBER OF YEARS SINCE DIAGNOSIS

	AGE ($\bar{x} \pm$ SD)	SEX(%) MALE	SEX(%) FEMALE	# years since diagnosis ($\bar{x} \pm$SD)
ALS-all	61.91 ± 8.79	52.6	47.4	2.85 ± 1.85
MG- all	53.59 ± 16.84	31.6	68.4	10.37± 8.066
MG ≥ 40y.o	59.33 ± 13.85			

TABLE 3 - PERCEIVED ILLNESS SEVERITY (%)

	EARLY	MODERATE	ADVANCED
ALS	15.8(3)	31.6(6)	52.6(10)
MG	15.8(3)	52.6(10)	31.6(6)

groups, and for this reason moderate and severe patients were compared separately. Some differences were noted in sex and years since diagnosis (Table 2). The ratio of males to females in MG was 0.46 whereas it was 1.11 in ALS. For this reason, the data was reanalyzed to control for sex by comparing sex-specific scores for all lifestyle variables. The mean number of years since diagnosis was greater for MG (Table 2). This could not be controlled for since there were only six MG patients in contrast to 18 ALS patients that were diagnosed five years ago or less. Race, marital status, income, and education were distributed relatively equally between the two groups (Tables 4-7). There was no relationship between the type of diagnosis and changes in employment status by Chi Square Analysis ($X^2 = 0.786$, $X^2 = 1.39$; NS).

Coping styles used by the two groups revealed a mean AC score that was greater for MG (68.40) than ALS (60.52) and a mean AB score that was greater for ALS (86.84) than MG (67.53). However, only the AB category was significant (T = 2.719, p < 0.05). The magnitude of the relationship remained the same when controlling for age, illness severity, and sex, however only the age-specific scores remained statistically significant (T = 2.381, p < 0.05). The lack of statistical significance probably reflects small sample size. MG and ALS patients both tended to be problem-focused (14/19 MG and 17/19 ALS) in dealing with their illness. Multiple T-tests were used to analyze these data due to small sample size. For this reason, these results must be applied with caution since the use of multiple T-tests increases the Type 1 error and the nominal significance level of 0.05 is not preserved.

Nonparametric Mann-Whitney U statistic was used to analyze the Cantril Ladder results for life satisfaction (LS), perceived health (PH), and social activity (SA). The MG median scores (7 for LS, 5 for PH, and 10 for SA) were higher than the ALS median scores (4 for LS, 4 for PH, and 1 for SA) in all three areas. For all three parameters there was a statistically significant association with type of diagnosis (Table 8). The strongest association was with social activity (p < 0.025). The relationship was

TABLE 4 - RACE (%)

RACE	MG	ALS
Caucasian	42.11(8)	52.63(10)
Asian	0	0
Black	36.84(7)	36.84(7)
Spanish American	15.79(3)	0
Other	5.26(1)	10.53(2)

TABLE 5 - MARITAL STATUS

	CURRENT		BEFORE DIAGNOSIS	
	MG	ALS	MG	ALS
Married	11	13	11	14
Widowed	4	1	1	1
Separated	0	3	1	2
Divorced	1	2	1	2
Single*	3	0	5	0

* (never married)

maintained when controlling for severity of illness, age, and sex, with the loss of statistical significance only for the moderate illness group, probably because the small sample size had a greater effect.

In internal LOC, the mean score was significantly higher for myasthenics than for ALS patients (T = 2.445, p < 0.05). The relationship was strongest in the advanced group (T = 2.165, p < 0.05). Age did not diminish the relationship (T = 2.117, p < 0.05). The magnitude of the relationship remained the same when controlling for sex, however the statistical significance of sex-specific scores was diminished, probably due to small sample size.

The myasthenic group scored significantly higher than the ALS patients in psychosocial functioning measured with the Likert scale (P < 0.01) (Table 9). The magnitude of all the relationships was upheld when controlling for age, sex, and severity of illness, although the moderate illness group failed to reach statistical significance and statistical significance was diminished in the male-specific group. Again, this was probably due to small sample size.

Fisher's Exact Probability test was applied to the public and body image

TABLE 6 - EDUCATION (%)

	MG	ALS
<9th Grade	21.05(4)	21.05(4)
10th Grade	5.26(1)	0
11th Grade	0	0
12th Grade	36.84(7)	26.32(5)
Vocational	10.53(2)	5.26(1)
Some College	21.05(4)	26.32(5)
College Graduate	5.26(1)	5.26(1)
Master's Degree	0	15.79(3)
Doctorate Degree	0	0

TABLE 7 - INCOME (%)

	MG	ALS
<$5,000	15.79(3)	21.05(4)
$5,000-10,000	42.11(8)	36.84(7)
$11,000-20,000	21.05(4)	10.53(2)
$21,000-30,000	10.53(2)	10.53(2)
>$30,000	10.53(2)	21.05(4)

TABLE 8 - LIFE SATISFACTION (LS), PERCEIVED HEALTH (PH), AND SOCIAL ACTIVITY
SCORES FOR PATIENTS WITH MG AND ALS. P values by Mann-Whitney U
nonparametric statistic.

	LS		PH		SA	
	U value	P(c)	U value	P(c)	U value	P(c)
All MGxALS	236.5	0.10	228.0	0.10	252.5	0.025
SEVERE MGxALS	71.5	0.001	80.0	0.001	69.5	0.001
MODERATE MGxALS	54.5	0.005	59.0	0.001	42.5	NS
MG ≥40yoxAll ALS	257.0	0.001	250.0	0.001	269.0	0.001
FEMALE MGxALS	86.5	0.05	103.0	0.001	82.5	0.100
MALE MGxALS	62.5	0.001	68.5	0.001	67.5	0.001

TABLE 9 - LIKERT T-SCORES AND P-VALUES FOR PSYCHOSOCIAL FUNCTIONING

	SOCIAL		PSYCH.	
	T score	P value	T score	P value
All MGxALS	3.951	<0.01	2.942	<0.01
SEVERE MGxALS	6.208	<0.001	2.616	<0.05
MODERATE MGxALS	0.510	NS	2.0516	<0.10
MG ≥40yoxAll ALS	3.162	<0.01	3.299	<0.01
FEMALE MGxALS	3.0307	<0.01	2.137	<0.05
MALE MGxALS	2.059	<0.01	1.484	<0.20

responses. A statistically significant relationship was established between type of diagnosis and both public and body image (Table 10). ALS patients consistently scored significantly higher than MG patients in terms of the number of questions to which they responded positively. Significantly more ALS patients than myasthenics hesitated to look in the mirror and felt that people were staring at them since their diagnosis. More ALS patients than myasthenics avoided public places. These relationships were maintained when controlling for age, sex, and severity of illness, and the decrease in statistical significance was again probably due to a diminution in sample size.

Myasthenics scored significantly higher than ALS patients on the QL index, a measure of QOL (T = 3.041, p < 0.01). The statistical significance remained when controlling for age (T = 3.000, p < 0.01), advanced illness (T = 2.619, p < 0.05), and male sex (T = 2.214, p < 0.05). Again, although the magnitude of all the relationships was upheld, statistical significance was diminished in both the moderate illness group and the female group.

DISCUSSION

Psychosocial problems often occur after receiving a diagnosis of a chronic or terminal disease. Numerous studies suggest that addressing the psychosocial aspects of long-term illness improves treatment outcome (Coates, Temoshok, and Mandel 1984; Zeldow and Pavlou 1984; Lok et al. 1985). However, past studies have indicated that psychosocial needs of patients with various life-long illnesses have not been sufficiently met. For example, Woo, Giardina, and Hilgartner (1985), in their cross-sectional study of B-thalassemia patients, found that patients' psychosocial needs were inadequately addressed in a hospital servicing the greatest number of B-thalassemia patients in the United States. There is a necessity to identify these needs early in order to alter the long-term outcome.

Investigators have repeatedly illustrated that intervention should take place early in order to be beneficial. Wiklund's longitudinal study showed that maladjustment two months after a myocardial infarction persists at one year (Wiklund et al. 1984). Oddy's longitudinal analysis of patients seven years after severe head injury showed little change in the psychosocial deficits since the two-year follow-up (Oddy et al. 1985). Robinson et al. (1985) assessed social functioning in stroke patients during the acute stroke period and at six months, and concluded that the most social intervention was needed during the initial stroke period to prevent withdrawal

TABLE 10 - PROPORTION OF PATIENTS WITH MG AND ALS RESPONDING POSITIVELY TO QUESTIONS. P values by Fishers Exact test.

	MG(%)	ALS(%)	P value(%)
I. BODY IMAGE			
hesitate to look			
in the mirror			
All MGxALS	10.53	42.11	1.59×10^{-9}
MG $\geq$ 40yoxAll ALS	6.67	42.11	5.38×10^{-9}
SEVERE MGxALS	16.67	60.00	9.99×10^{-4}
MODERATE MGxALS	10.00	33.33	5.00×10^{-4}
FEMALE MGxALS	7.69	33.33	1.01×10^{-5}
MALE MGxALS	16.67	50.00	8.74×10^{-4}

TABLE 10 (continued)

II. PUBLIC IMAGE feel that people are staring at them			
All MGxALS	21.053	42.11	2.25×10^{-8}
MG ≥40yoxAll ALS	20.00	42.11	1.25×10^{-7}
SEVERE MGxALS	16.67	60.00	9.99×10^{-4}
MODERATE MGxALS	20.00	33.33	1.37×10^{-3}
FEMALE MGxALS	23.077	44.44	1.29×10^{-4}
MALE MGxALS	16.67	40.00	7.49×10^{-4}
If yes, does this cause them to avoid public places?			
All MGxALS	25.00	50.00	1.212×10^{-2}
MG ≥40yoxAll ALS	50.00	50.00	4.44×10^{-2}
SEVERE MGxALS	0.00	33.33	1.43×10^{-1}
MODERATE MGxALS	50.00	100.00	6.67×10^{-1}
FEMALE MGxALS	33.00	50.00	1.14×10^{-1}
MALE MGxALS	0.00	50.00	2.00×10^{-1}

and social isolation. Similar findings for amputation patients were obtained by Parkes (1975).

According to the literature, the concept of LOC might improve the success of education and treatment groups for long-term medical problems. Wallston et al. (1976) studied the responses of obese females to one of two randomly assigned weight reduction programs: a self-directed program (internally oriented) and a group program (externally oriented). External LOC patients tended to lose more weight in the group program whereas internals lost more weight in the self-directed program (Wallston et al. 1976; Wallston and Wallston 1978).

Coates, Temoshok, and Mandel (1984) studied AIDS patients and found that psychosocial factors may increase susceptibility to chronic and infectious diseases, influence the disease course, and contribute to health-promoting or health-damaging behavior. Both Deyo et al. (1983) and Liang and Jette (1981) emphasized that in chronic disease, such as rheumatoid arthritis, management should be directed toward preservation of psychosocial and physical function. It has been suggested that defense mechanisms and coping behaviors influence the course of the disease (Coates, Temashok, and Mandel 1984; Heim, Moser, and Adler 1978; Bloom and Spiegel 1984).

ALS patients had a significantly higher AB coping score than myasthenics, possibly because they could not intellectually justify why they had this disease and instead reverted to overt behavioral attempts to deal with the problem and its effects. In contrast, MG patients had a greater AC coping score, as well as a significantly higher internal LOC score. Perhaps because there is no treatment for their illness, ALS patients are more reluctant than myasthenics to consider themselves able to influence the disease course. MG patients, in contrast, may know from past experience that their symptoms can partially be alleviated by taking the right drug or resting at the proper time. These results can be applied to redesigning programs and services by providing self-directed programs for internal LOC patients and group programs for externals, since it has been shown that patients tend to do better in programs compatible with their own LOC (Wallston et al. 1976; Wallston and Wallston 1978; Schulman 1979).

The higher scores for MG patients in life satisfaction, perceived health, social activity, and QOL is consistent with Brown's study which showed that social activity was the most important factor in life satisfaction and that an individual's own perception of his health is the most significant predictor of well-being (Brown, Rawlinson, and Hilles 1981). The ALS patients' worse public and body image than the myasthenics not only supports Purtilo's (1976) notion that distorted public and body image occurs in chronic and terminal illness, but also suggests that these changes are more severe in terminal than chronic disease.

The similarity of MG and ALS allows generalization of these results to the larger population of the chronically and terminally ill. Future studies comparing other chronic and terminal diseases that also have internal consistency might add to the knowledge base. Some difficulties encountered using ALS and MG, such as the lack of a younger subgroup for ALS patients and the rapidity of disease progression with ALS as compared to MG, might be better controlled when comparing other diseases. Additional information could be obtained from a longitudinal design that studies patients from the onset of diagnosis and follows them with serial questionnaires.

This study provides important preliminary data showing that adjustment needs of the chronically and terminally ill differ. The knowledge that these differences exist and the ability to detect them is important in light of the vast literature indicating that early intervention minimizes long-term problems and maladjustment influences the disease course. Knowing that the chronically and terminally ill each have their own distinct psychosocial stresses will allow services to be more specifically targeted. Not only will this promote more cost-efficient and productive use of available services, but the goal of alleviating maladjustment, withdrawal and social isolation, and incapacitation will be more readily achieved. The form used in this study, or a modified version, could be used for high-risk screening. Programs, services, and guidelines for staff training may need to be reorganized. The results of this study should be used as a basis for continued and more extensive research.

CONCLUSION

The findings of this study suggest that differences exist between the effects of treatable and untreatable diagnoses on lifestyle that may warrant different kinds of psychosocial support. Specifically looking at the two diseases used to study the larger hypothesis, it was found that MG patients did better in all areas than ALS patients. They scored significantly higher in life satisfaction, perceived health, social activity, psychological adjustment, and QOL. MG patients had a significantly better public and body image than ALS patients. Adjustment patterns differed in that ALS patients used AB coping more than MG patients, whereas MG patients used internal LOC more than ALS patients. A survey form, which was modified from previous questionnaires in the literature, was able to detect these differences. This suggests the usefulness of a short survey form in the ambulatory setting to periodically assess patients in order to follow their adjustment and to see if their psychosocial needs are being met. In this way, adequate health care can more effectively be provided to an ever-increasing proportion of our society—the chronically and terminally ill.

REFERENCES

Billings, A. G. and R. H. Moos. 1981. "The Role of Coping Responses and Social Resources in Attenuating the Stress of Life Events." *Journal of Behavioral Medicine* 4(2):139-157.

Bloom, J. R. and D. Spiegel. 1984. "The Relationship of Two Dimensions of Social Support to the Psychological Well-Being and Social Functioning of Women with Advanced Breast Cancer." *Social Science and Medicine* 19(8): 831-837.

Brown, J. S., M. E. Rawlinson, and N. C. Hilles. 1981. "Life Satisfaction and Chronic Disease: Exploration of a Theoretical Model." *Medical Care* 19(11):1136-1146.

Charles, R. A. 1985. "Coping with Life on a Portable Ventilator." *Home Health Care Nurse* 3(2):27-30.

Coates, T. J., L. Temoshok, and J. Mandel. 1984. "Psychosocial Research is Essential to Understanding and Treating AIDS." *American Psychology* 39 (11):1309-1341.

Corney, R. H. and A. W. Clare. "The Construction, Development, and Testing of a Self-Report Questionnaire to Identify Social Problems." *Psychology of Medicine* 15:637-649.

Deyo, R. A., T. S. Inui, J. D. Leininger, and S. S. Overman. 1983. "Measuring Functional Outcomes in Chronic Disease: A Comparison of Traditional Scales and a Self-Administered Health Status Questionnaire in Patients with Rheumatoid Arthritis." *Medical Care* 21(2):180-192.

Forsyth, G. L., K. D. Delaney, and M. L. Gresham. 1984. "Vying for a Winning Position: Management Style of the Chronically Ill." *Research in Nursing Health* 7(3):181-188.

Heim, E., A. Moser, and R. Adler. 1978. "Defense Mechanisms and Coping Behavior in Terminal Illness." *Psychotherapy and Psychosomatics* 30:1-17.

Holahan, C. J., and R. H. Moos. 1981. "Social Support and Psychological Distress: A Longitudinal Analysis." *Journal of Abnormal Psychiatry* 90(4):365-370.

Janiszewski, D. W., J. T. Caroscio, and L. H. Wisham. 1983. "Amyotrophic Lateral Sclerosis: A Comprehensive Rehabilitation Approach." *Archives of Physical and Medical Rehabilitation* 64:304-307.

Liang, M. H. and A. M. Jette. 1981. "Measuring Functional Ability in Chronic Arthritis." *Arthritis and Rheumatism* 24(1):80-86.

Lok, A. S. F., D. J. Van Leeuwen, H. C. Thomas, and S. Sherlock. 1985. "Psychosocial Impact of Chronic Infection with Hepatitis B Virus on British Patients." *Genitourinary Medicine* 61:279-282.

McFarlane, A. H., G. R. Norman, D. L. Streiner, R. Roy, and D. J. Scott. 1980. "A Longitudinal Study of the Influence of the Psychosocial Environment on Health Status: A Preliminary Report." *Journal of Health and Social Behavior* 21:124-133.

Mulder, D. W., E. H. Lambert, and L. M. Eaton. 1959. "Myasthenic Syndrome in Patients with Amyotrophic Lateral Sclerosis." *Neurology* 9(10):627-631.

Muscular Dystrophy Association. 1984. *Amyotrophic Lateral Sclerosis* (Pamphlet).

Muscular Dystrophy Association. 1986. *Myasthenia Gravis Fact Sheet* (Pamphlet).

Myasthenia Gravis Foundation. 1985. *Myasthenia Gravis: A Manual for the Physician.*

Myasthenia Gravis Foundation. 1986. *Facts about Myasthenia Gravis for Patients and Family* (Pamphlet).

Oddy, M., T. Coughlan, A. Tyerman, and D. Jenkins. 1985. "Social Adjustment After Closed Head Injury: A Further Follow-up Seven Years After an Injury." *Journal of Neurosurgery* 48:564-568.

Parkes, C. M. 1975. "Psychosocial Transitions: Comparison Between Reactions to Loss of a Limb and Loss of a Spouse." *British Journal of Psychiatry* 127:204-210.

Purtilo, R. B. 1976. "Similarities in Patient Response to Chronic and Terminal Illness." *Physical Therapy* 56(3):279-284.

Robinson, R. G., P. L. Bolduc, K. L. Kubos, L. B. Starr, and T. R. Price. 1985. "Social Functioning Assessment in Stroke Patients." *Archives of Physical and Medical Rehabilitation* 66(8):496-550.

Schipper, H. and M. Levitt. 1985. "Measuring Quality of Life: Risks and Benefits." *Cancer Treatment Report* 69(10):1115-1122.

Schulman, B. A. 1979. "Active Patient Orientation and Outcomes in Hypertensive Treatment Application of a Socio-Organizational Perspective." *Medical Care* 27(3):267-280.

Sivak, E. D., W. T. Gipson, and M. R. Hanson. 1982. "Long-Term Management of Respiratory Failure in Amyotrophic Lateral Sclerosis." *Annals of Neurology* 12:18-32.

Spitzer, W. O., A. J. Dobson, J. Hall, E. Chesterman, J. Levi, R. Shepherd, R. N. Battista, and B. R. Catchlove. 1981. "Measuring the Quality of Life of Cancer Patients: A Concise QL Index for Use by Physicians." *Journal of Chronic Diseases* 34:585-597.

Udaka, F., S. Yamao, H. Nagat, S. Nakamura, and M. Kameyama. 1984. "Pathological Laughing and Crying Treated with Levodopa." *Archives of Neurology* 41:1095-1096.

Wallston, B. S., K. A. Wallston, G. D. Kaplan, and S. A. Maides. 1976. "Development and Validation of the Health Locus of Control (HLC) Scale.'' *Journal of Consulting Clinical Psychology* 44(3):580-585.

Wallston, B. S. and K. A. Wallston. 1978. ''Locus of Control and Health: A Review of the Literature.'' *Health Education Monographs* 6:107-117.

Ware, J. E. 1984. ''Conceptualizing Disease Impact and Treatment Outcomes.'' *Cancer* 53:2316-2323.

Wiklund, I., H. Sanne, A. Vedin, and C. Wilhelmsson. 1984. ''Psychosocial Outcome One Year After a First Myocardial Infarction.'' *Journal of Psychosomatic Research* 28(4):309-321.

Wilson, R. W. and Drury, T. F. 1984. ''Interpreting Trends in Illness and Disability: Health Statistics and Health Status.'' *Annual Review of Public Health* 5:83-106.

Zeldow, P. B. and M. Pavlou. 1984. ''Physical Disability, Life Stress, and Psychosocial Adjustment in Multiple Sclerosis.'' *Journal of Nervous and Mental Disorders* 172(2):80-84.

Living with Amyotrophic Lateral Sclerosis (ALS)

Richard F. Mayer

The Neuromuscular Service at the University of Maryland Hospital in Baltimore, Maryland was established to investigate, diagnose, and manage patients with a number of different neuromuscular diseases. Many of these diseases result in partial or complete muscular paralysis and, therefore, disable the patient. Diseases such as myasthenia gravis and the Guillain-Barre syndrome, which can cause generalized paralysis, are treatable, and most patients can recover even from respiratory paralysis (Sellman and Mayer 1985; Koski, Khurana, and Mayer 1986). Other disorders such as hereditary hypertrophic polyneuropathy and adult onset muscular dystrophy or atrophy may be very slowly progressive and patients can lead active, productive lives. Although many of the neuromuscular disorders do disable patients, amyotrophic lateral sclerosis (ALS) stands out as the most disabling of the whole group, with the poorest prognosis. In recent drug trials in ALS, we became acutely aware of how disabling and hopeless this disease really is from the patient's standpoint (Potes et al. 1986) (Figure 1). The drug trials were aimed at trying to better understand and to alter the function of motor neurons-units in these patients. However, as the disease progressed in all the patients studied, we became more involved in helping patients to live with ALS.

In order to better understand the patients' and the families' feelings about ALS and how it had altered their lives, interviews and questionnaires were used to obtain this information. This report summarizes the data obtained, emphasizing how patients live with this progressive terminal disease.

Richard F. Mayer, MD, is Professor of Neurology and Director of Neuromuscular Service, The University of Maryland School of Medicine, Baltimore, MD 21201.

FIGURE 1. Clinical status of ALS patients determined by a neurological exam and score (NE); zero is a normal NE and 15 is complete paralysis of cranial and extremity muscles. Note the continued progression of the weakness in all groups of patients studied and treated over 18 months.

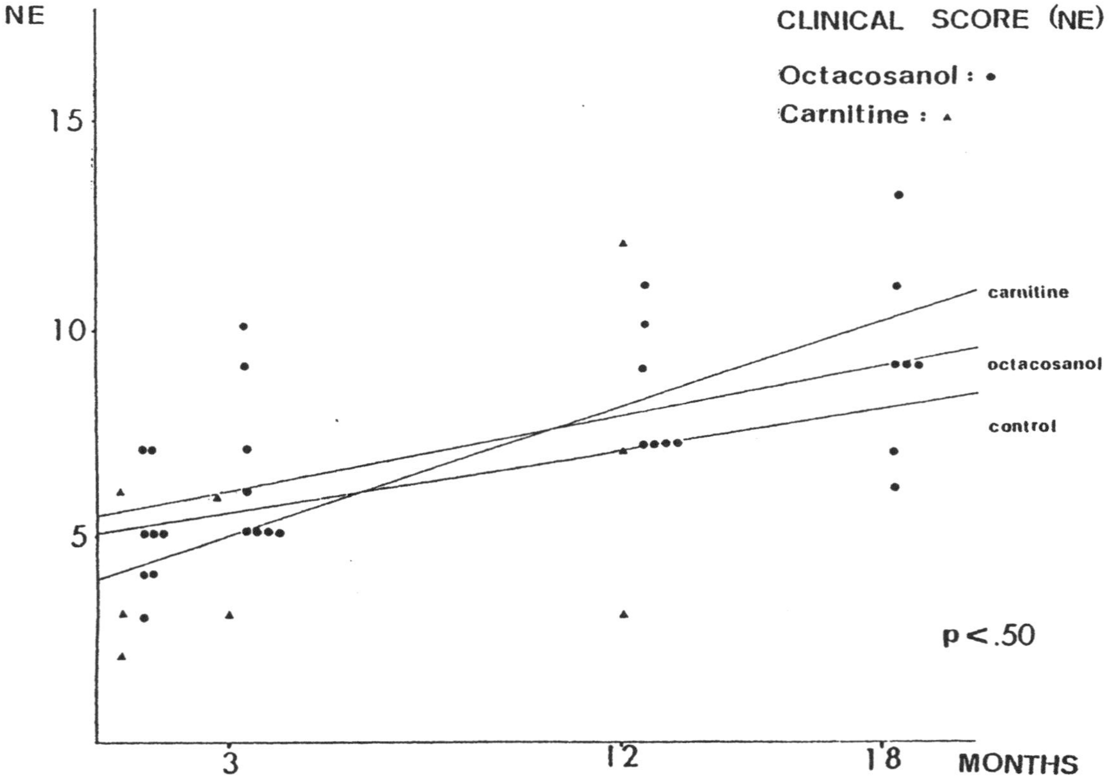

24

CLINICAL MATERIAL

The diagnosis of ALS was established by neurologic examinations, electrophysiological studies, neuroimaging, and, in some, myelograms, cerebrospinal fluid analysis, and muscle biopsies. Thirty-three patients (42 percent males, 58 percent females, mean age of 59 years, range 29 to 81) were studied and followed beginning in 1982 (Table 1). Of these, 76 percent have died during the study period. The surviving patients have mild to moderate weakness, all continue to become weaker, and none have improved.

Group I, consisting of 8 patients, received a 24-month trial of octacosanol, a long-chain alcohol found in wheat germ oil; Group II, consisting of 5 patients, received a 23-month trial of oral L-carnitine (Sigma Tau), that is essential in long-chain fatty acid metabolism in nerve and muscle; Group III, 6 patients, received vitamins and supportive care during this period; and Group IV, 15 patients, received varied treatments following the conclusion of the study of Groups I to III.

Interviews with patients, families, and friends were carried out during their visits to the Neuromuscular Clinic. Questionnaires were sent to patients and families. These included questions on how the diagnosis was made and relayed to them; their understanding of the disease; concerns about the progression and prognosis; how they were managing and coping with the progressing disability; its impact on their lives, futures, and family; and what type of terminal care they wanted, including their feelings about a living will.

RESULTS

Results of the interviews and questionnaires are summarized in Table 2 and as follows. The diagnosis was often withheld (in 30 percent), guessed by the patient, relayed by the family, or "crudely done" by a physician (in 30 percent). In one patient, the wrong diagnosis was initially established and a surgical procedure done. Both patients and families were greatly upset by the diagnosis of ALS and its prognosis. They usually received little support from the physician, but were able to obtain help from others such as friends, support groups, and religious personnel.

With the diagnosis of ALS established, the main concerns of the patients were: becoming disabled and dependent on others (in 50 percent). The length of the illness, the type of progression, and the terminal phase were also of concern. The families had the same concerns but felt helpless watching the progression of the disease and the paralysis. They had con-

TABLE 1. ALS Patient Data

TREATMENT	SEX	AGE YEARS	DURATION MONTHS	SURVIVAL
OCTACOSANOL	5M 3F	31-75 (55)	30-78 (51)	25%
L -CARNITINE	3M 2F	45-69 (62)	12-90 (59)	40%
VITAMINS	1M 5F	57-70 (63)	7-90 (37)	17%
VARIED	6M 9F	29-70 (54)	7-72 (32)	27%

TABLE 2. Summary of Interview and Questionnaire Results

INITIAL DIAGNOSIS

PATIENT

EXPECTED, GUESSED DIAGNOSIS

WITHHELD, CRUDELY DONE

ANXIETY OF DISEASE

WRONG DIAGNOSIS

FAMILY

UPSET BY DIAGNOSIS

LITTLE SUPPORT FROM MD

EMOTIONAL IMPACT

MAIN CONCERNS

PATIENT

BEING DISABLED, DEPENDENT

LENGTH OF ILLNESS, PROGRESSION

FAMILY

MENTAL AND PHYSICAL STRESS

COMFORT, FINANCIAL NEEDS

TABLE 2 (continued)

HOW COPING

PATIENT

HELP FROM FAMILY

AGENCIES, MANAGING

DEVASTATED LIFE

FAMILY

ABLE TO HELP, STRESSFUL

PROVIDE PHYSICAL AND

EMOTIONAL SUPPORT

TERMINAL CARE

PATIENT

LIMITED SUPPORT THERAPY

COMFORTABLE, AT HOME

PHYSICAL AIDS

FAMILY

SHORT TERM IF POSSIBLE

EXPERIMENTAL THERAPY

LITTLE HELP FROM PSYCHIATRY

cerns for the patient's emotional as well as physical status, and they tried to make the patient as comfortable as possible. Financial concerns were always present but were minor compared to the other problems.

As the disease progressed, the patients and families appeared to manage. Their lives were devastated, however, and some families disintegrated (15 percent). Most families worked together to help the patient and provided the essential emotional and physical support (60 percent). As one husband said, "For me it was tough because she was at home until she passed away. I took care of her at night and on weekends. However, no matter how bad it became for me, I could not feel sorry for myself because what was happening to her was so cruel that my life, as bad is it was, was great by comparison. It's an overwhelming psychological problem for those doing the caring as well as the one suffering." However, all of the patients were depressed and they expressed concern over their progressing paralysis and eventual death. Help from agencies and support groups was available and helpful to many of the patients and especially to the families.

The terminal phase of the illness varied in length. Most patients and families preferred limited medical support, without invasive therapy, at home (60 percent). Several patients established living wills to prevent invasive therapy. Most did not wish to be cared for in hospital or hospice and preferred to remain at home (80 percent). However, physical aids and experimental drugs were requested by most. At this stage most patients and families wanted and needed medical support but few felt psychiatrists were of much help. Some stated that religious personnel were especially helpful. Families requested that the terminal phase be as short and painless as possible, while some of the patients hesitated or declined to answer this question (20 percent). Most patients were prepared for the terminal phase and were able to accept it more readily than their families.

DISCUSSION

In any medical-neurologic discussion of how patients live with ALS, we usually first consider all the possible physical aids to help the individual become more independent, and then second, all the pharmaceuticals that make them more comfortable. These are available to patients with ALS and help family and patient cope with the disease and disability. However, they may not be sufficient to help the patient adjust to a progressive, paralyzing, lethal disease. A number of drugs are also helpful in the treatment of anxiety, fear, and depression of ALS patients. Families, friends, religious personnel, and support groups were found to be the most helpful to the emotional state of these patients. Most of the patients did manage with their families, and the terminal illness helped pull most families together, but it did shatter a few. From observing these patients, it appears that those who accepted the disease as a terminal one managed the best. It is likely that an individual's acceptance of his or her mortality is the first step in dealing with such a disease. However, varied family and home situations made it possible for some to cope better with ALS. Providing the emotional support, along with physical aids and drugs, was helpful to most patients and families. Helping them to remain active in their work or hobby was also helpful to many. The home environment was especially important to most. It should be possible to maintain most ALS patients at home during the terminal phase of the illness. Only a few patients were admitted for terminal care, either because of severe pain or the family's inability to deal with a dying loved one. This was usually dealt with and prepared for by the family before the terminal phase. Most families handled this well. Dying over a period of time is the expected course of ALS and facing this aspect of the disease is most important for neurologists and all those involved with the patient's care. Keeping the patients comfortable and at home with their families during the terminal phase seems the best approach at the present time.

SUMMARY

ALS is a progressive paralyzing disease without known etiology or treatment that results in death. The duration of the disease varies with the localization and extent of paralysis, and few patients survive after five years of neurologic signs. Patients and families need to deal with the emotional and physical stress of this disease, as do physicians and members of society. Patients can live with a progressive disabling disease such as ALS, be productive, and yet be prepared for death. It is important for us to improve the support services and groups that provide the physical, emotional, and terminal help for patients with ALS.

REFERENCES

Koski, C. L., R. Khurana, and R. F. Mayer. 1986. "Guillain-Barre Syndrome." *American Family Physician* 34:198-210.

Potes, E., S. Cherry, P. M. Hoffman, and R. F. Mayer. 1986. "Therapeutic Trials in Amyotrophic Lateral Sclerosis." *Muscle and Nerve* 9(5S):140.

Sellman, M. S. and R. F. Mayer, 1985. "Treatment of Myasthenic Crisis in Late Life." *Southern Medical Journal* 78:1208-1210.

Family Response
to Duchenne Muscular Dystrophy

Jessica Robins Miller

Duchenne muscular dystrophy (DMD) is a chronic, relentlessly progressive disease that requires multidimensional medical, rehabilitative, and psychosocial management. Individuals do not exist within a vacuum. The presence of a child or young adult with Duchenne dystrophy in a family seriously affects the family unit as a whole. Although this essay will focus on family response to Duchenne muscular dystrophy, many of the comments will be relevant to other progressive diseases as well.

Mattsson (1977) defines coping as adaptational techniques used by an individual to master a major psychological threat and its attendant negative feelings in order to achieve personal and social goals. Coping with muscular dystrophy presents a unique set of challenges to both individuals and their families.

Much of the literature on coping and adjusting to chronic illness and physical disability discusses various stages that individuals and families move through (Pearse 1977; Bray 1980; Drotar, Baskiewicz, Irvin, Kennell, and Klaus 1975; Vaughn and Mendell 1986). Authors discuss emotional responses to crisis (denial, shock, anger, and grief), and state that individuals and families must move through a set of stages before they reach a phase of acceptance. While different authors discuss different emotional patterns, there is general agreement that once this process has been completed, one has adjusted to the disability crisis or loss. The stages of adjustment are also discussed in the grief and loss literature (Kübler-Ross 1969). However, based on extensive clinical experience, family adjustment to Duchenne muscular dystrophy does not occur in this

Jessica Robins Miller, ACSW, LICSW, is Social Work Consultant at Massachusetts Hospital School in Canton, MA and is also in private practice.

31

pattern. While families may experience common emotions and feelings, they adjust and respond in individual ways. Personality, prior experiences, and the meaning the family attributes to the diagnosis all have a bearing on how they will react. It is important not to lock families into expected reaction categories, but rather to listen to their differences as well as their similarities. Not all families feel the same thing at the same time, nor do they adjust in the same manner.

Case Report

When discussing reaction to diagnosis in a parent support group, Mr. H stated that he became very angry and depressed, and remained so for many months. Mr. T, on the other hand, described his adjustment period as lasting one weekend. Upon returning from the doctor's office, Mr. T locked himself in a room with a bottle of Scotch, dealt with all his feelings and emotions and then moved on with his life.

Neither of these fathers adjusted more or less effectively than the other. Each one moved through a process that was unique to him. Not only do families adjust differently from one another, within a family unit it is not uncommon for individual members to experience different emotions at different times, intensities, and rates.

Case Report

Soon after learning that their son had muscular dystrophy, Mr. and Mrs. C entered counseling. Mr. C stated that he had been very depressed since they had received the diagnosis, and angry with his wife for not feeling depressed along with him. Through exploration it was determined that within their relationship, Mr. and Mrs. C rarely were depressed at the same time. In the past, when one got depressed the other remained in the supportive and strong role. Mrs. C was therefore afraid that if she too became depressed, they would not survive the crisis. Discussing this together helped the C's to feel more connected with each other, rather than alone and isolated with their feelings.

Adjustment to muscular dystrophy never stops. It is an ongoing, fluctuating process in which developmental changes and the progressive nature of the disease interface with each other repeatedly. With each developmental stage the child reaches, the family must incorporate the disability and resulting limitations. Concerns and challenges that arise within each developmental phase present the family with a new experience. Due to the progressive nature of the disease, the family repeatedly encounters a series of losses that are both physical and emotional in nature. Therefore it is helpful to view the adjustment process as a series of conflicts and resolutions surrounding periods of change and loss, as distinct from a pattern with a beginning and end point such as described in the "stage theory" of adjustment. While families may come to terms with the initial diagnosis and subsequent lifestyle, they must continue to adjust to loss throughout the course of the disease.

The process of adjusting to muscular dystrophy is complex in that it has elements of adjusting to acute disability (since the child is usually not diagnosed until age two or older), chronic disability (the child will always have it), progressive disability (it will get worse), and terminal disease. Over the years many stresses will surface, some phases more difficult to cope with than others. Clinical experience has shown that the following four time periods offer the most challenges to families, with multiple conflicts to be resolved: diagnosis, cessation of ambulation, adolescence, and the late stages of the disease.

DIAGNOSIS

The diagnosis of muscular dystrophy represents a crisis to the family. Parad and Caplan (1966) define crisis as an upset in the steady state of equilibrium caused by a hazardous event that creates a threat, a loss, or a challenge to the individual. Family systems theory states that individual family members hold different roles within the family unit, and equilibrium is maintained when all roles function in conjunction with each other. When a crisis occurs, families experience a period of disequilibrium, as they become immersed in a situation they were not adequately prepared to handle. When working with families it is important to recognize that crisis is time limited, that it is not a psychiatric disorder, and that some families grow as they work through the crisis. However, during a crisis period, familiar coping stategies may not work, leaving the family feeling ineffectual. In addition, old losses may surface that have not been thoroughly worked through, making this a very trying time for the family.

Case Report

Shortly after Mrs. M learned about her son's diagnosis, she was hospitalized for severe depression. In the hospital, it was discovered that as an adolescent, Mrs. M had witnessed her brother's death after he was hit by a car. Mrs. M's family was so devastated by the event, their only means of coping was to not talk about it. They forbade Mrs. M to talk about it as well. Mrs. M, left to deal with the loss on her own, did so by blocking it out. The threatened loss represented by the diagnosis of DMD caused Mrs. M's previous loss to surface, resulting in acute depression. Mrs. M had to work through her feelings related to her brother's death before she could begin to deal with her current loss.

Upon learning about the diagnosis of muscular dystrophy, many families experience feelings of loss and threat as well as fear and anxiety related to the prognosis (Mattsson 1977). Denial is not uncommon during this period. Families may deny the existence, the impact, or the permanence of the disability. They may accept the diagnosis, but deny the permanence. Denial can be a healthy process and should not be interfered with in the early stages. Snyder (1988) discusses beneficial denial as a process that may allow an individual to tolerate an unpleasant reality that cannot be changed, and thus enable effective functioning. Gossler (1987) defines healthy denial as a task of balancing hope and despair, denial and acceptance.

Case Report.

Mary, a physical therapist, recognized the signs of Duchenne muscular dystrophy in her son two years before she brought him to a neurologist for an evaluation. Looking back several years later she remarked, "I knew he had muscular dystrophy, and even though my pediatrician encouraged me to have him evaluated, I could not bring myself to do it. Nor could I share my suspicions with my husband. I had to deny what was happening so that I could enjoy those years. I knew what was ahead for him and for us once the diagnosis was confirmed."

The conflict of the diagnostic period revolves around the crisis of the diagnosis. Families need to react, grieve, and respond while maintaining a balance in the family system. Family members also need time to mourn the loss of the expected healthy child. New dreams can be built, but not until old ones are buried.

CESSATION OF AMBULATION

It is helpful to view cessation of ambulation as a process rather than as an endpoint. This is a very stressful time for families as they become immersed in a state of limbo for an extended period of time. It begins when the child first exhibits difficulty ambulating and ends when the child begins to use the wheelchair full time. During this time, the child is neither able bodied nor fully wheelchair dependent. Most children experience a period of tripping and falling, often leading to emergency room visits. The conflict arising during this period is when and how to introduce the wheelchair. Family members question whether offering the wheelchair will decrease the motivation to walk. In addition, the wheelchair signifies the child's progressive weakness, which can be devastating for the family. However, to not intervene is also difficult for the family as they become increasingly concerned about the child's safety.

When the concept of the wheelchair is introduced early, it allows the child and family time to adjust. Some families prefer to keep a manual wheelchair in school in case of fatigue or long distances, before the child requires it on an ongoing basis. When the child becomes fully wheelchair dependent, the transition can be eased if he is provided with a motorized wheelchair, which allows more mobility and more independence. At this point, the family often experiences mixed feelings representing loss and relief. While wheelchair dependency is dreaded by the family, in retrospect many view it as a more positive time than anticipated for two reasons. One, it ends a prolonged period of limbo which has been quite stressful, and two, many families discover that they have been preparing for the wheelchair for many years, easing the adjustment process.

Case Report

In counseling sessions, Mrs. M discussed her depression in the context of her son's birthdays. Tom was 8, yet Mrs. M remembered clearly the prediction that her son would be in a wheelchair by the time he was 10. Each birthday, therefore, represented a closer step to the time when her child would not be able to walk, and caused Mrs. M to feel very sad. When Tom finally did begin to use the wheelchair, Mrs. M found it much less difficult to cope with than she had anticipated. She realized she had actually been adjusting to this loss since Tom was diagnosed.

Although many families find the transition to the wheelchair easier than expected, it is crucial to recognize and acknowledge this to the family as a major loss.

ADOLESCENCE

Adolescence is a stressful time for most individuals and their families. For the family who has a disabled child it can be especially trying, as it is a time when differences are acutely felt. Adolescence raises many conflicts regarding independence and dependence. For the child with muscular dystrophy, the constant conflict of adolescence revolves around striving to be independent at the same time that his physical condition is deteriorating, causing a more dependent status. Similarly the family is pulled into a more dependent role (providing the physical needs) at a time when they should be letting go and establishing a more independent relationship with their child. Several additional factors come into play that intensify this relationship during the adolescent years. When the child enters junior high school he is separated from his peer group of the elementary years and begins to form new relationships. The individual with DMD may find this quite difficult, especially if he is struggling with adjusting to the wheelchair at the same time. Parents often discuss the loneliness of their children, and their efforts to fill weekends with activities that will involve them. For the socially involved adolescent, activities tend to revolve around his house due to its accessibility, and transporting to and from activities falls to his family because of the accessible van. Some adolescents and families struggle with this ongoing dependent status at a time when both of their peer groups are becoming more independent. One of the major tasks of adolescence is separation from the family. With Duchenne muscular dystrophy, separation needs to be conceptualized within the framework of progressive disease.

Case Report

In a parent support group Mr. O talked about his abundance of activities with his 16-year-old son, and his lack of activities with his wife and friends. When the issue of separation was brought up Mr. O stated, "If I'm only going to have my son for a few more years, why shouldn't I spend as much time with him as possible."

Another area of conflict arising for the family during adolescence is sexuality. Siegel and Kornfeld (1983) define sexuality as the evolution of sexual feelings and self-identity, socially and physically. It is difficult for family members to see their disabled child as a sexual being as this brings to the surface additional emotions, fears and concerns. Due to the anticipated shortened life span, many families do not think about their children engaging in typical adolescent behaviors such as dating or drinking. Therefore, when these issues come up, the family is faced with additional stresses.

Case Report

Mrs. T arrived home one afternoon to find her 16-year-old son drinking with his friends. Never having faced the situation before, her concerns and outrage stemmed from two sources. She was worried about her son's safety, thinking about the possibility of his falling out of his wheelchair while drunk. She was also flooded with feelings about adolescence and drinking behavior. She stated that she never anticipated having to deal with this issue and it was just one more thing to worry about. On some level Mrs. T had hoped she could avoid the whole matter.

LATE STAGE OF THE DISEASE

No matter how well a family has prepared for the late stage of the disease, it is often one of the most frightening and difficult periods. The child or young adult with DMD is often uncomfortable, has difficulty sleeping, and begins to have respiratory involvement. For the parents, it is a time when they are beginning to question their own independence, as they observe the children of their friends moving on for educational or vocational pursuits. In addition, death and dying issues become paramount for families as they feel the presence of death more acutely. As boys graduate from their local high schools, friends move away; new relationships are often difficult to make, leaving the individual more alone. The family feels more isolated as well, as the personal care needs of the child or young adult take up increasing amounts of time, and getting out of the house becomes more difficult. Visits to the muscular dystrophy clinic become fewer, as families often feel there is little more that can be done for them. The conflicts during this period are twofold: First, families struggle to maintain hope, while living with the realities of impending death. Some people feel guilty over wishing for death to come as a relief from pain and suffering. Second, if offered a choice, families face the complex decision regarding ventilator support.

For persons with muscular dystrophy, the concept of extending life with a ventilator remains controversial, and protocols for decision making and initiating use are inconsistent (Miller, Colbert, and Schock 1988). When family members are provided with the choice, the decision is complex. Most families are informed at the time of diagnosis that life expectancy will be short, and although this is painful, on some level they have come to terms with that fact by the time ventilator decisions must be made. In addition, family members arrive at this juncture following many years of caring for a progressively dependent child. They are often exhausted, yet have incorporated a routine system of care provision into their lives. The ventilator adds an additional limitation on an already limited life. The option of extending life presents the family with a psychological dilemma, as they are faced with preparing for a future they were told would not exist. Many families seriously consider the decision to let the disease take its natural course. However, a family may feel that they are signing their child's death certificate if they opt against ventilator support. If a decision needs to be made quickly, parents are put in the position of alleviating or prolonging their child's suffering. It is not surprising that, when given the option, most families choose ventilation.

When options are provided, questions are raised regarding the decision-making process, as this decision moves beyond the boundaries of medicine, reaching into the parameters of economy, ethics, and the law. For example, who is the primary decision maker? If consensus cannot be reached, who has the right to make the final decision: the patient, the family, the physician, or an outside source? One advantage of the decision-making process in progressive disease is the time available for patients and families to make an educated and prepared decision, as opposed to traumatic onset disability where life support is provided on an emergency basis. The time inherent in a progressive illness should enable patients and families to make informed and timely decisions, yet to date few protocols provide a systematic approach to decision making with optimal planning time. Decisions to extend life with a ventilator belong to the patient and family. Health care providers can assist by educating and counseling and by providing support and permission for either choice.

TASKS FOR ADJUSTMENT

Throughout the progression of the disease, there are many tasks for adjustment for both the individual and the family. Some of these include: understanding the physical limitations of the disease, becoming familiar with the necessary personal care and medical management (which changes with the progression of the dystrophy), striving to be as independent as possible within the confines of dependency, and discovering ways to compensate. Two of the major tasks in the adjustment process for the family are expressing feelings and mastering stress. The adjustment process is facilitated when family members are able to express their feelings regarding the disease process. However, this can often be frightening and overwhelming. Family therapy can be very useful in helping family members express such emotions.

Case Report

The S family came into family therapy when their son Bob was 10. Even though Bob had been diagnosed with DMD when he was two, the S family had been unable to share the news with Mr. S's parents. Mrs. S's brother had DMD, and her family was aware of the diagnosis. Feeling that they could no longer hide the truth, the S family felt they had to tell Mr. S's family but did not know how to go about it. When exploring the issue, it became clear that Bob and Mrs. S both had a lot of unresolved feelings about hiding the truth.

Bob was convinced he had something so terrible that if his grandparents knew about it, it would kill them. Mrs. S was exhausted from the energy spent hiding her son's deteriorating condition. Neither one of them understood Mr. S's reasons for not telling his family, and were both feeling angry. Mr. S had been unable to tell his family because he felt that, as long as they didn't know the truth, Bob would not really have muscular dystrophy. Therefore, informing his family of the diagnosis meant that Mr. S could no longer deny it, which frightened him greatly.

Family therapy enabled the S family to express their feelings, thereby increasing their understanding of each other's reactions and concerns and allowing them to deal with the sadness of the diagnosis together, rather than individually.

Mastering stress is another difficult task for adjustment. In addition to the areas already mentioned, stress experienced by families stems from several sources: witnessing their child's pain and discomfort, knowing the disease can be hereditary, being concerned about siblings, having to explain the disease to others, and negotiating systems (school, medical, social, and financial).

CHALLENGES

In addition to dealing with the initial crisis of the diagnosis and all subsequent crisis periods and conflicts throughout the course of the disease, the challenges for families are many. There is coping and adjusting to role changes while maintaining a balance within the family system, responding to questions, decision making and defining and planning for the future.

In addition to filling the traditional roles of mother and father, parents become nurses, therapists, educational managers, financial managers, advocates, and sometimes sole sources of emotional support. Filling these roles makes it difficult to maintain an equilibrium in the family system. Family members are often balancing quality time with care providing time. Regarding a home physical therapy program, one mother remarked:

> By the time you get home from work, make dinner, deal with homework and baths, doing exercises is the last thing you want to be doing. And, if the choice is spending quality time with him or doing exercises that make him uncomfortable, there doesn't seem to be much choice, does there?

This attitude seems to be more prevalent among families with older children. If the child is still ambulating, family members will carry through an exercise program with the hopes that it will make a difference. Most families do reach a point when they abandon the program, but not without a certain amount of guilt. Relationships between the disabled child and his siblings, and the siblings and the parents, also require balances. If there are a number of household tasks that need to be completed, and it is impossible for the disabled child to complete them, the nondisabled child is likely to have more to do. Furthermore, time with the parents may be shortchanged due to the disabled child's excessive personal care needs. The effects of a disabled child on the siblings does not appear to be all negative, however. Many families feel that the nondisabled siblings have had a positive growth experience as a result of their situation. Time alone as a couple also needs to be negotiated but unfortunately often drops to the bottom of the priority list. Couples need permission to spend time together, away from their children.

Responding to a child's questions presents the family with an enormous challenge. Some of the questions these parents are asked include: Why does this happen to me? Will I get better? If I go to therapy will the disease go away? If therapy isn't helping and it hurts, why do you do it? If I have surgery will I be cured? Am I going to die?

Within the context of trying to maintain hope while living with progressive disease, these are very complex questions. Family members need time to discuss and process them before they are called upon to answer them.

Families of DMD individuals are faced with complex decision-making challenges throughout the course of the disease. From the time of diagnosis, families are faced with decisions without clear-cut answers. Some of the dilemmas facing families concern:

- diagnosis and prognosis—when and how much to tell the child and other family members;
- cessation of ambulation—when and how to introduce the wheelchair;
- exercise and surgical interventions. They may be risky and do not halt the progression of the disease, but they may prolong the onset of what is to come;
- educational activities—whether to mainstream or segregate the adolescent; and
- ventilator support—whether to extend life or let the disease take its natural course.

Permission for all options is crucial after education is provided regarding choices, procedures, risks, and expected benefits.

Defining and planning for the future is become more and more of a challenge as ventilator options and age of life expectancy are changing. How do you plan for the future when you are unsure of what the future will be? Many families learn to live on a day-to-day basis early in the course of the disease. However, some phases of the disability require longer term planning.

There are many intervention strategies from which families who have children with muscular dystrophy can benefit. An initial goal is to help the family see the child as a child first, and a child with a disability second. All members of the health care team can be of assistance by listening, problem solving, providing education, and including the family as a team member. Specific psychosocial interventions are also useful. Based on a thorough assessment, these may include the following: crisis intervention, a brief treatment modality focusing only on the current crisis; family counseling, which assists the family (without the disabled child present) in adjusting to the disability and related changes; family therapy, which involves working with the disabled child and family together and removes the concept of the identified patient; and group therapy.

In conclusion, family adjustment to muscular dystrophy is a complex process that is ongoing and fluctuating. Families do not all adjust and respond in the same manner; yet many experience common emotions and feelings. Duchenne muscular dystrophy is a devasting event for any family. Understanding the psychosocial issues and challenges, in addition to the course of physical deterioration, is essential for all professionals who work with this patient population.

REFERENCES

Bray, G. P. 1980. "Rehabilitation of Spinal Cord Injured: A Family Approach." In P. W. Power and A. E. Dell Orto, eds. *Role of the Family in the Rehabilitation of the Physically Disabled*. Baltimore, MD: University Park Press.

Drotar, D., A. Baskiewicz, N. Irvin, J. Kennell, and M. Klaus. 1975. "The Adaptation of Parents to the Birth of an Infant with Congenital Malformation: A Hypothetical Model." *Pediatrics* 56:710-717.

Gossler, S. 1987. "A Look at Anticipatory Grief: What is Healthy Denial." In L. I. Charash, R. E. Lovelace, S. G. Wolf, A. H. Kutscher, D. P. Roye, C. F. Leach, eds. *Realities in Coping with Progressive Neuromuscular Disease*. Philadelphia: Charles Press.

Kübler-Ross, E. 1969. *On Death and Dying*. New York: MacMillan.

Mattsson, A. 1977. "Long-Term Physical Illness in Childhood: A Challenge to Psychosocial Adaptation." In R. H. Moos, ed. *Coping with Physical Illness*. New York: Plenum Medical Book Company.

Miller, J. R., A. P. Colbert, and N. C. Schock, 1988. "Ventilator Use in Progressive Neuromuscular Disease: Impact on Patients and Families." *Developmental Medicine and Child Neurology* 30(2):200-207.

Parad, H. J. and G. Caplan. 1966. "A Framework for Studying Families in Crisis." In H. J. Parad, ed. *Crisis Intervention: Selected Readings*. New York: Family Service Association of America.

Pearse, M. 1977. "The Child with Cancer: Impact on the Family." *The Journal of School Health* March, 1977: 174-178.

Siegel, I. and M. S. Kornfeld. 1983. "Parent Support Group in the Management of Duchenne Muscular Dystrophy: A Combined Medical and Psychosocial Approach." In L. I. Charash, S. G. Wolf, A. H. Kutscher, R. E. Lovelace, and M. S. Hale, eds. *Psychosocial Aspects of Muscular Dystrophy and Allied Diseases: Commitment to Life, Health, and Function*. Springfield, IL: Charles C. Thomas.

Snyder, R. D. 1988. "On the Use of Denial." In M. Lazarus, D. J. Cherico, H. N. Melore, A. H. Kutscher, R. Halporn, and A. M. Bregman, eds. *Muscular Dystrophy and Allied Diseases: Perspectives on Psychosocial Issues, Selected Papers*. New York: Archives of the Foundation of Thanatology.

Vaughn, A. J. and J. R. Mendell. 1986. "Maternal Attitudes and Adjustments to Terminal Illness in Duchenne Muscular Dystrophy." In L. I. Charash, A. Bregman, E. R. Prichard, R. E. Lovelace, A. H. Kutscher, and J. Kelemen, eds. *Muscular Dystrophy and Allied Diseases: Impact on Patients, Family and Staff*. New York: The Foundation of Thanatology.

Psychosocial Issues and Case Management in Myotonic Muscular Dystrophy

Marcia Sirotkin-Roses

Myotonic muscular dystrophy (DM) is the most prevalent form of muscular dystrophy. Steinert (1909) described it as a slowly progressive disease that initially affects the distal musculature with weakness and atrophy. Facial muscles are also involved, causing the "myotonic facies," a hatchet-like appearance, often in conjunction with alopecia. This disease can progress to involve the proximal muscles and may cause severe ambulation difficulties that require the patient to use a wheelchair for mobility. Clinically, myotonia is the difficulty of the muscle to relax. Myotonia is demonstrated as sustained deplorization (dive bomber effect) on electromyogram (EMG) (Davison 1961; Lipicky and Bryant 1973) and by percussion on clinical exam (Appel and Roses 1978; Harper 1979).

Other organ systems are involved as well. Cardiac abnormalities in the form of conduction delays may cause loss of consciousness or even total heart block (DeBacker et al. 1976; Griggs et al. 1975; Lambert and Fairfax 1976; Payne and Greenfield 1963) which can lead to sudden death. A proband case may present with multisystemic involvement including hypothyroidism, fertility problems, and diabetes mellitus (Appel and Roses 1978; Roses, Harper, and Bossen 1979). Swallowing difficulties, abdominal pain, hyper-somnolence, and presenile iridescent cataracts are also common (Garrett et al. 1969; Davison 1961; Coccagna et al. 1975; Fleischer 1918; Hughes et al. 1965; Klein 1958). However, the diagnosis is not always clear cut, as the proband may present with few symptoms and no weakness or muscle stiffness, making the link between these symptoms

Marcia Sirotkin-Roses, LP, MA, is Research Associate, Division of Neurology, and Assistant Professor, Department of Physical Therapy, Duke University Medical Center, Durham, NC 27706.

The author wishes to thank Donna Surdyka-Just, MSW, for her assistance with the questionnaire and Dorothy Gentry and Ginger Tuck for their secretarial assistance.

43

difficult to realize. DM does have a variable genetic expressivity and penetrance, and some heterozygotes with the disease show no clinical involvement at all (Adie and Greenfield 1923; Bundey, Carter, and Soothill 1970; Roses 1985). EMG and slit lamp examination are helpful tools, but patients may never get tested with these if the diagnosis of DM is not suspected or if the symptoms are not ocular or neuromuscular in nature. Certainly many patients are missed by family history. Therefore, if there is evidence of DM in a proband, his family should be screened as well (Bundey, Carter, and Soothill 1970; Polgar et al. 1972). The Duke Neuromuscular Research Clinic (NMR) and the Duke MDA Clinics have been following this course for the past 13 years. We now follow over *500* patients with DM in North Carolina. These families have contributed to the physiologic, biochemical, and molecular genetic data that have lead to the ability we have today to detect heterozygotes with high accuracy (Bartlett et al. 1987; Miller, Roses, and Appel 1976; Pericak-Vance et al. 1986).

Mental slowness has long been recognized as characteristic in many patients with DM (Harper 1979; Rosman and Kakulas 1966; Thomasen 1948). Klein (1958) and Caughey and Myrianthopoulos (1963) found apathy and the lack of initiative among the personality quirks they noted most frequently in their DM patients. Also, they stated that the severity of muscle weakness seemed to correlate to the degree of mental impairment in their patients. However, no formal IQ or psychometric testing was instrumented (Strub and Black 1977). Of course, most of the congenital myotonic dystrophy patients are born floppy and are severely retarded. Sixty-eight percent of Harper's congenital DM population had mental retardation, whereas only 12 percent of his DM patients from a series of 170 initially presented with mental impairment (Harper 1975, 1979).

The cause of central involvement has been investigated by many. Some related it to the high frequency of hypersomnolence, which in turn was related to hypoventilation in these patients (Coccagna et al. 1975). Others postulated an increased incidence of inclusions in the thalamic nuclei of DM patients (Culebras, Feldman, and Merk 1973). At this time conclusive data for a central deficit is still unknown.

In addition, there are known, expected personality characteristics. We in the Duke NMR clinics have noted a reticent, suspicious, or even hostile nature in our patients on field visits to their homes, giving us limited cooperation from them initially. Also, some have severe dysarthria which impairs oral communication. A combination of apathy, mental slowness, or hypersomnolence also blurs an accurate medical history. They deny or fail to recognize the existence of their symptoms, and it is necessary to depend on their normal spouse, relatives, or caretakers to assist with this.

These same characteristics lead to the social deterioration seen in many patients with DM (Caughey and Myrianthopoulos 1963; Roses 1973; Sirotkin-Roses 1983). These patients fail to cope with ordinary daily living events. Their socioeconomic level is lower than that of their normal siblings (Sirotkin-Roses 1983) and often to a degree greater than their physical involvement can explain. When placed in the mainstream of social function or employment, they are unable to maintain the placement level (Roses 1973; Sirotkin-Roses 1983). They gradually lower their daily functional level to simple tasks around the home or to watching TV and sleeping most of the day. They are a self-limiting, self-isolated population.

I have already mentioned the variable expressivity of this disease. Though autosomal dominant, DM can manifest later in life with few symptoms and no impairment early on (Roses 1985). There are few in our DM population who have reached high socioeconomic levels. Their mental capacity was unimpaired. About a dozen attended university or were schooled beyond a high school education. A few have become professionals or administrators. Almost all of these have had to withdraw gradually from full participation at their original entry level. Case IA (see patient data) is an LPN who is now unable to turn a patient in bed due to weakness nor give hypodermic injections due to myotonia in his hands. However, most of our patients were only able to enter the work force as unskilled laborers or blue collar workers. Also, a good number entered the armed forces and served before they became symptomatic. In addition, those impaired at an earlier age, manifesting symptoms in their late teens and early twenties, usually never become employable at a high level, drop out quickly (Case II B), or lack the initiative to seek employment at all. The combination of their physical impairment, their apathy, and mental impairment is a strong block against integration into the normal socioeconomic stream.

Ninety percent of our DM patients live in a rural community. In these smaller towns there are fewer referral agencies to assist a handicapped individual. Also, there are fewer jobs available and less variety. The lifestyle is less varied than in an urban region. However, the daily activities of the 38 DM individuals who participated in the survey do not reflect those of the general rural North Carolina population. Fourteen of these DM individuals watch TV or rest during most of the day. Five help with yard work, six do some housework, five sleep often. Four subjects do some form of recreational activity or exercise (walk, fish, bike ride, hunt), but only seven work (one additional man works a nightshift). Fifty percent of the 38 subjects with myotonic dystrophy do nothing during the day (Table 1).

A few subjects are frustrated and angry that their physical impairment has hampered their previous abilities (e.g., jogging or hunting — Subject IVB and IVC). Four others are upset that they are no longer the breadwinner. Two claim their disease led to their divorces, and only three are fearful that this disease might affect their children in a similar way. But, the majority (70 percent) are content. The upward mobility of this population is to a large extent self-limiting.

Many handicapped individuals in North Carolina manage to obtain financial assistance, home health aides, physical or speech therapy, transportation to clinics, and social services. The Duke MDA clinics are directed toward helping these patients obtain the services they need. Also, there are local support groups to assist families with the problem of chronic illness, however, only one family in our entire DM clinic population has joined a support group. Also many DM patients do not follow through with service provider's suggestions. DM individuals tend to neglect themselves, making this disease one of the least addressed in total patient care. We realize their educational and occupational levels are dependent on the degree of their impairment, but on a daily basis, how independent are these individuals? Could they do more?

A survey was mailed to 71 randomly chosen adult patients with myotonic muscular dystrophy. Thirty-eight patients responded. The survey requested limited socioeconomic information and a checklist for helpfulness of services the patients might use. Each of the 38 subjects received a follow-up interview. Fourteen of the patients could not complete the questionnaire due to manual dexterity difficulties or to poor comprehension. They were assisted by a relative or caretaker. Six patients required assistance during the interviews due to dysarthria or to limited knowledge of their financial support system. The medical history of each subject was reviewed for socioeconomic data.

The survey and interviews revealed information about the interactions these patients had with various providers. Personality conflicts were prominent in eight individual interactions. In general, physicians, physical therapists, and social workers were the most helpful providers, but not all patients required the use of each of these. However, social workers were also the least helpful. They were the most frustrating to deal with, followed by psychologists and vocational rehabilitation counselors. The

TABLE 1. Activities of DM Subjects

#Patients	Daily Activities
14*	TV/Rest
5	Yard Work
6	Housework
5*	Sleep often
4	Recreational activity
7	Work
1	Works a night shift (sleeps all day)

19* DM subjects (50% are inactive on a daily basis).

MDA clinic was the most helpful agency with 35 positive responses, though bias is surely present here. Other helpful agencies were social services (9 +), SSI (8 +), church (7 +) and mental health services (5 +).

Part III of the survey required additional descriptive information. Twenty patients answered the first question — how have the services been helpful — with most referring to equipment they received. Only 12 answered any of the remaining questions. These last questions and the interviews were most informative in defining each individual's unmet needs or problems. For example, six patients required additional financial assistance.

The 38 participants divided into three distinct groups. Nine are self-supporting. Two of these are employed and unmarried and the seven others manage on either retirement funds or SSI. The survey revealed there are 10 individuals who are supported entirely by relatives or caretakers and 20 who are supported by relatives and their own government supplements. Two of these 20 do try to work at part-time employment as a babysitter or in summer construction. These 30 supported individuals range in age from 19 to 63 years.

Table 2 demonstrates that the employed subjects with DM are still not self-supporting. This list does not include the 10 patients who worked at a time previous to this survey; six of these were in the armed forces, one was an RN and one a banker (both retired by 50 years old) and two were part-time employees.

There are 100,000 people with myotonic muscular dystrophy in the United States. How far should society go to support this population beyond benefits that already exist? The DM patients in our clinic are seen more often than many and are well-assisted by the clinic personnel. The MDA supports myotonic muscular dystrophy as one of many dystrophies. Certainly there are not many other advocates for this disease. The general population is not worried about contracting DM as it would AIDS. It is not as devastating as other genetic diseases such as Duchenne muscular dystrophy or neuromuscular diseases such as amyotrophic lateral sclerosis, or late onset diseases such as Alzheimer's disease. The DM population does not advocate for itself; there is no political lobby. Indeed, the general population is usually unaware of myotonic muscular dystrophy. However, these individuals do need assistance.

The caretaker's role in many chronic diseases becomes one of financier, daily aide, chauffeur, social worker and advocate. In DM this is demanding to the extent that some caretakers must spend full time with the affected individual (patient IIIA). The majority of the moderately affected

TABLE 2

AGE	MALE	FEMALE	MARITAL STATUS	SELF-SUPPORTING
29	LPN		S	N
32	Sheltered Workshop		S	N
34	Sheltered Workshop		S	Y
35	Fireman		M	N
49		Receptionist	M	N
34	Night Watchman		S	N
38		Lab. Technician	M	N
35	Salesman		S	Y

individuals cannot live alone—some are too weak or too somnolent to perform simple everyday tasks. Others would sleep through meals, whereas some with dysarthria need assistance to eat. The question is not just how society can help the affected individual with a chronic illness, but should we not also consider training the caretakers in an extended caretaker network. This role model is most visible in the Alzheimer's Disease Support Network, a nationwide program. Through the interview sessions it became obvious that the caretakers are anxious to join support groups and learn how to manage respiratory infections, heart problems, and swallowing disorders. They would like to eliminate falls in relatives and, especially, they would like to eliminate this disease and prevent future generations from getting it.

We can best help the myotonic muscular dystrophy population by counseling these caretakers. If a family is screened early enough, caretakers can help guide their children into proper classroom situations and later into sensible, nonphysical employment. Awareness of medical symptoms and signs could, perhaps, prevent some cases of sudden death, especially in families with a known history of arrhythmias. Most important is the knowledge gleaned from genetic counseling that can be passed through the family.

The availability of linkage markers makes heterozygote detection quite accurate in DM (Bartlett 1978). With linkage techniques in informative families there is a 99 percent accuracy of diagnosis. This is clinically significant for future generations as well as in the prenatal diagnosis of congenital DM. As many clinicians are aware, it is usually the normal wife of an affected husband who will present for prenatal diagnosis even though she is at little risk for offspring with congenital DM. The affected females who are at risk for congenital DM children present a genetic testing and counseling problem which is indeed characteristic of the DM population in general (Schrott, Karp, and Omenn 1973). They may show disinterest, poor comprehension, or reticence and hostility. It is more probable that these counseling efforts will reach the DM population through the efforts of clinically unaffected siblings or the normal family members, the caretakers. In our clinic the largest demand for genetic screening has been by clinically asymptomatic siblings of affected individuals who want confirmation that they are not heterozygotes and can proceed with their families without worry. These individuals could be counseled to advocate for genetic screening of their families with the knowledge that clinical care of patients can be extended to relatives in order to determine gene carrier diagnosis.

REFERENCES

Adie, W. J. and J. G. Greenfield. 1923. "Dystrophia Myotonica (Myotonia Atrophica)." *Brain* 46:73-127.

Appel, S. H. and A. D. Roses. 1978. "Muscular Dystrophies." In J. B. Stanbury, J. B. Wyngaarden, and S. Fredrickson, eds. *The Metabolic Basis of Inherited Disease.* New York: McGraw Hill, pp. 1260-1281.

Bartlett, R. J., M. A. Pericak-Vance, L. H. Yamoka, J. R. Gilbert, M. Herbstreith, W. Y. Hung, J. E. Lee, T. Mohandas, G. Bruns, C. Laberge, M. C. Thiabult, D. Ross, and A. D. Roses. 1987. "A New Probe for the Diagnosis of Myotonic Muscular Dystrophy." *Science* 235:1648-1650.

Bundey, S., C. O. Carter, and J. F. Soothill. 1970. "Early Recognition of Heterozygotes for the Gene for Dystrophic Myotonica." *Journal of Neurology, Neurosurgery and Psychiatry* 33:279-293.

Caughey, J. E. and N. C. Myrianthopoulos. 1963. *Dystrophia Myotonica and Related Disorders.* Springfield, IL: Charles C Thomas.

Coccagna, G., M. Mantovani, C. Parchi, F. Mironi, and E. Laugaresi. 1975. "Alveolar Hyperventilation and Hypersomnia in Myotonic Dystrophy." *Journal of Neurology, Neurosurgery and Psychiatry* 38:977-984.

Culebras, A., R. G. Feldman, and F. Merk. 1973. "Cytoplasmic Inclusion Bodies Within Neurons of the Thalamus in Myotonic Dystrophy: A Light and Electron Microscopic Study." *Journal of Neurological Science* 19:319-329.

Davison, S. I. 1961. "The Eye in Dystrophia Myotonica, with a Report on Electromyography in the Extra-ocular Muscles." *British Journal of Ophthalmology* 45:183-196.

DeBacker, M., P. Bergmann, A. Perissino, P. Gotignies, and R. J. Kahn. 1976. "Respiratory Failure and Cardiac Disturbances in Myotonic Dystrophy." *European Journal of Intensive Care Medicine* 2:63-67.

Fleischer, B. 1918. "Uber Myotonische Dystrophie Mit Katarakt." *Albrecht v. Graefes Arch. Ophthal.* 96:91-133.

Garrett, J. M., T. D. Dubose, J. E. Jackson, and J. R. Norman. 1969. "Esophageal and Pulmonary Disturbances in Myotonia Dystrophica." *Archives of Internal Medicine* 123:26-32.

Griggs, R. C., R. J. Davis, D. C. Anderson, and J. T. Dove. 1975. "Cardiac Conduction in Myotonic Dystrophy." *American Journal of Medicine* 59:37-42.

Harper, P. S. 1975. "Congenital Myotonic Dystrophy in Britain. Part I. Clinical Aspects." *Archives of Diseases of Childhood* 50:505-513.

Harper, P. S. 1979. *Myotonic Dystrophy.* Philadelphia: W. B. Saunders.

Hughes, D. T. D., J. C. Swann, J. A. Gleeson, and F. I. Lee. 1965. "Abnormalities in Swallowing Associated with Dystrophia Myotonica." *Brain* 88:1037-1042.

Klein, D. 1958. "La Dystrophie Myotonique (Steinert) et la Myotonic Congenitale (Thomsen) en Suisse: Etude Clinique Genetique et Demographic." *Journal Genetica Humana* 7:1-328.

Lambert, C. D. and A. J. Fairfax. 1976. "Neurological Associations of Chronic Heart Block." *Journal of Neurology, Neurosurgery, and Psychiatry* 39:571-575.

Lipicky, R. J. and S. H. Bryant. 1973. "A Biophysical Study of the Human Myotonias." In J. E. Desmedt, ed. *New Developments in Electromyography and Clinical Neurophysiology.* Basel: Karger, pp. 451-463.

Miller, S. E., A. D. Roses, and S. H. Appel. 1976. "Scanning Electron Microscopy Studies in Muscular Dystrophy." *Archives of Neurology (Chicago)* 33:172-174.

Pericak-Vance, M. A., L. H. Yamoka, R. F. Assinder, W. Y. Hung, R. J. Bartlett, J. M. Stajich, P. C. Gaskell, D. A. Ross, S. Sherman, G. H. Fey, S. Humphries, R. Williamson, and A. D. Roses. 1986. "Tight Linkage of Apolipoprotein C2 to Myotonia Dystrophy on Chromosome 19." *Neurology* 36(11):1418-1423.

Polgar, J. G., W. G. Bradley, A. R. M. Upton, J. Anderson, J. M. L. Howat, F. Petit, D. F. Roberts, and J. Scopa. 1972. "The Early Detection of Dystrophia Myotonica." *Brain* 95:761-776.

Roses, A. D. 1985. "Myotonic Muscular Dystrophy: From Clinical Description to Molecular Genetics." *Archives of Internal Medicine* 145.

Roses, A. D., P. S. Harper, and E. H. Bossen. 1979. "Myotonic Muscular Dystrophy." In P. J. Vinken and G. W. Bruyn, eds. *Handbook of Clinical Neurology.* New York: Noah Holland Publishing Company, Vol. 40, pp. 485-532.

Roses, M. J. 1973. *Social and Physical Variables in Myotonic Muscular Dystrophy.* Doctoral dissertation, University of North Carolina, Chapel Hill, NC.

Rossman, N. P. and B. A. Kakulas. 1966. "Mental Deficiency Associated with Muscular Dystrophy: A Neuropathological Study." *Brain* 89:769-788.

Schrott, H. G., L. Karp, and G. S. Omenn. 1973. "Prenatal Prediction in Myotonic Dystrophy: Guidelines for Genetic Counseling." *Clinical Genetics* 4:38-45.

Sirotkin-Roses, M. J. 1983. "Myotonic Dystrophy: Social Variables." In L. Charash, S. G. Wolf, A. H. Kutscher, R. E. Lovelace, and M. S. Hale, eds. *Psychosocial Aspects of Muscular Dystrophy and Allied Diseases.* Springfield, IL: Charles C. Thomas,, pp. 101-121.

Strub, R. L. and F. W. Black. 1977. *The Mental Status Examination in Neurology.* Philadelphia: F. A. Davis Co.

Steinert, H. 1909. "Uber das Klinische und Anatomische Bild des Muskelschwunds der Myotoniker." *Dtsch. Z. Nervenheilk* 37:58-104.

Thomasen, E. 1948. *Myotonia. Thomsen's Disease, Paramyotonia and Dystrophia Myotonica: A Clinical and Heredobiological Investigation.* Copenhagen: Munksgaard.

APPENDIX. Patient Data

AGE	EMPLOYED	BILLS COVERED BY	DAILY ACTIVITY
38	N	Friend/VA disability	TV, read
29	Y*	Parents/Pt	Work
40	N	Relatives	TV, yard
29	N	Parents/SSI	Rest, yard, fish
58	N	Spouse/VA	TV, rest
19	N	Parent	TV
32	N	Parents	Yard, rest
62	N	Spouse, SSI	Yard, rest
40	N	SSI	Rest
43	N	Spouse	House
34	N	Spouse/Stock dividends	Rest, read
51	N	Spouse/summer pt. employment	TV read
32	Y*	Parent	Work
48	N	Parent	
52	N	Retirement pension/SS	Read
60	N	Caretaker/SS	TV, rest
32	N	VA	TV, hunt
63	N	Spouse/SS	
31	N	Parent	TV, babysit, bike
58	N	Spouse/SSI/VA	TV, read
39	N	Spouse/SS	House
34	Y*	PT/SSI	Work
46	N	Retirement fund/SSI	House, read

35	Y*	Spouse/PT	Work
49	Y*	Spouse/PT	Work
48	N	SS/SSI	TV
30	Y*(P/T)	Spouse/SSI/PT	Work, house
31	N	SSI/SS	
34	Y*	Parent/PT	Sleeps, works nights
39	N	Spouse	House, childcare
32	N	SS	TV, house
35	Y*	PT	Work
48	N	Parent/SSI	TV, sleep
57	N	Spouse/VA	
42	N	Parent	TV
24	N	Relative/SSI	
42	N	Spouse/SSI	House
46	Y*	Spouse/PT	Work

Patient

IA   29-year-old male employed as a floor LPN, lives with parents.
     Diagnosis at 25 with mild distal and proximal weakness, myotonic facies
     and percussion myotonia on clinical exam plus EMG in 1986. Has mild
     dysphagia and hypernasal speech.

IIA 40-year-old male lives at home with adopted parents. Was in sheltered
     workshop for a short time but fatigued. Now cares for pets at home.
     Has severe distal weakness and mild proximal, moderate dysarthria and
     facial weakness. Wears bilatral AFO's last 2 years. Missed many
     clinic appointments. 1st degree AVB.

IIIA 58-year-old male. Diagnosis in 1965. At home with wife who cannot work
     since care for husband is so demanding over last year. Patient is
     wheelchair bound for last 1 1/2 years. No muscle grades greater than
     grade 3. 1st degree AVB, PR interval > 2 (Ventricular premature
     complex, left anterior fasicular block, left ventricular hypertrophy).
     Severe dysarthria. 1983 KAFO braces but unable to use now. Mild
     dysphagia-liquids and solids. Needs functional hand splints. County
     Social Services to supply respite care. Patient also has diabetes and
     cataracts.

IIIB 32-year-old male works in sheltered workshop, but has been too fatigued for last month - job became hazardous. Diagnosis at 12 years old. Now with moderated dysarthria, facial weakness, steppage gait and dysphagia since 1983. 1st degree heart block since 1975. Lives at home with parents. Wears AFO's.

IIIC 31-year-old female lives at home with parents. Never employed full-time. Part-time babysitting this year. Dropped by Vocational Rehabilitation for disinterest. Diagnosis at 11 years old. Now has mild dysarthria and facial weakness. Good general muscle strength in extremities. Mild goiter. Hysterectomy at 30 years old. EKG within normal limits. Rides bicycle.

IVA 60-year-old male. Fifth grade education, was in armed forces. Diagnosis at VA in 1963. First noticed weakness at 25 years old. Did not work after discharge. 1960 cardiac arrhythmia, 1966 swallowing difficulty and lingual myotonia. Now bilateral ptosis, severe dysarthria, dyspnea, testicular atrophy, post 2x cataract surgery and bilateral detached retina. Falls 6x week during transfers. Walks only few steps - uses tricart. Cannot self-fed or dress. 1983 pacemaker implant, second degree heart block. Rule out CHF-patient has nocturnal dyspnea and ankle swelling.

IVB 31-year-old male with eleventh grade eduation. At 14 years old noticed action myotonia. Never did well in school academically or in athletics. Two incidents of chest pain in high school: Diagnosis of mitral valve prolapse. Now steppage gait - uses AFO's. Nasal speech, unilateral ptosis, myotonic facies. Status post bilateral cataract removal. Some yard work, hangs around house, fishes, sleeps, reversed sleep pattern frequent.

IVC   33-year-old male likes to hunt, but cannot lift up gun and requires special trigger and vehicle hunt permit. In process of divorce. Depressed (post ETOH, drugs). Abnormal and excessive sleep pattern. Mild dysarthria and dysphagia (lingual myotonia). PAC's and PVC's, 1983 RVH. Numerous respiratory infections. Spent 4 years in Navy after high school and took 3 years of classes at technical school— stopped secondary to financial difficulties.

QUESTIONNAIRE

PART I. INSTRUCTIONS: PLEASE COMPLETE THIS QUESTIONNAIRE AND MAIL IT
BACK TO US IN THE ENCLOSED ENVELOPE BY MONDAY JUNE 29, 1987. THANK YOU.

Your Name _____ Age _____
Person filling out this form (if other than self) _____
What is your major source of income? _____

Are you employed? _____ If yes, where? _____

Who lives in your house? _____

Who pays the household bills? _____

What activities fill up most of your time during the day? _____

PART II. INSTRUCTIONS: PLACE A CHECK MARK ON THE APPROPRIATE LINE TO
SHOW IF THE AGENCIES AND PERSONS LISTED BELOW HAVE HELPED YOU OR NOT.

AGENCY AND PROVIDERS	HELPFUL	NOT HELPFUL	NEVER USED
DEPT.OF SOCIAL SERVICES			
Choreworker	____	____	____
Social Worker/Caseworker	____	____	____
CHURCH ASSISTANCE			
Pastor	____	____	____
Church Members/Volunteers	____	____	____

58

COUNTY HEALTH DEPARTMENT
Physician
Social Worker
Visiting Nurse

HOME HEALTH AGENCY
Home Health Aide
Visiting Nurse
Physical Therapist
Social Worker

MDA CLINIC
Physician
Physical Therapist
Social Worker
Genetic Counselor
Equipment Vendor

MENTAL HEALTH CENTER
Psychiatrist/Psychologist
Social Worker
Family Counselor

SCHOOL/EDUCATIONAL CENTER
Principal
Teacher
Guidance Counselor
Physical Therapist
Speech Therapist

QUESTIONNAIRE (continued)

	HELPFUL	NOT HELPFUL	NEVER USED
SOCIAL SECURITY ADMIN.			
Intake Worker	___	___	___
Social Worker/Caseworker	___	___	___
TRANSPORTATION SERVICES			
Driver Education Instructor	___	___	___
Bus/Van/Taxi Driver	___	___	___
Motor Vehicle Policeman	___	___	___
DEPT. VOCATIONAL REHABILITATION	___	___	___
Vocational Counselor	___	___	___
Rehab. Engineer	___	___	___

PART III. INSTRUCTIONS: PLEASE ANSWER THE FOLLOWING QUESTIONS:

In what ways have these services and people been most helpful to you and your family? _____

_____

_____

60

In what ways have these services and people not been helpful?

_____
_____
_____

How might services be improved for you and your family?

_____
_____
_____

If you use services not found on this form please list them.

_____
_____
_____

Muscular Dystrophy: Assessing the Impact of a Diseased State

Michael K. Bartalos

Recently we witnessed two major breakthroughs in our understanding of muscular dystrophy: the exact location of the gene for the Duchenne and Becker types of muscular dystrophy has been located, and the gene product, a long-sought-after protein, has been identified. These discoveries are major milestones in our understanding of the disease and harbor the hope for finding rational therapy for muscular dystrophy in the not-too-distant future. For the time being, however, curative treatment is still a distant goal and symptomatic treatment remains our only alternative.

The nature of the interaction between physicians and other health care professionals on one hand, and the patient and his or her family on the other, is best observed in the course of a prolonged illness with a hopeless outcome. Muscular dystrophy and several other genetic diseases, along with many forms of cancer and AIDS, are examples of such illnesses. The prolonged course of the illness calls for a long-term relationship between health care providers and the patient and family. This relationship is subjected to strains and trials caused by changes in the patient's health status, psychological changes, and often by changes in economic conditions.

The family that is struggling to come to terms with the approaching loss might have difficulty financing the care called for and might be physically exhausted by the long hours of extra duty spent in the care of the ill family member.

The patient who is bewildered by his or her condition might be depressed and angry at the hopelessness of the situation, or horrified by what Carl G. Jung (1965) described as "the slow, irresistible approach of the

Michael K. Bartalos, MD, is Assistant Professor of Clinical Pediatrics, College of Physicians and Surgeons, Columbia University, and Director, Institute for Genetic Medicine, New York, NY 10032.

63

well of darkness which will eventually engulf everything you love, possess, wish, strive, and hope for.''

The health care professionals are frustrated by the continuous decline of the patient's health despite their best efforts. They are impatient with the ineffectiveness of their art, and they might — at some dark moment — question the utility of their efforts. Nowhere is the underlying assumption or philosophy of illness and care better displayed than in situations where a near-crisis atmosphere prevails over a prolonged period of time.

HUMAN INTERACTIONS

Man is a complex system of interacting parts functioning as a whole. He interacts with his environment as a unit. This environment includes objects, subjects, and concepts. In our activities we fill a physical, economic, and emotional void. When we are sick, our functioning is altered and our interaction with others is altered. Our actions are altered, which provokes altered reactions from others. Thus our illness, our recovery, our death is bound to affect those around us.

In our interaction with the environment and others we fulfill one of these roles: sustaining (being an asset); neutral (being an incidental); extenuating (being a burden). Thus at any given time in our interaction with another person we can be perceived as an asset, an incidental or a burden. The concepts of asset and burden have two parameters, namely duration and intensity, while incidental has one, duration.

Interaction between two persons represents a series of actions and reactions. If we introduce a third person into this equation, the interaction becomes more complex. With three persons interacting, we can envision a situation where a person is perceived simultaneously as an asset by one and as a burden by the other. It can also happen that all three perceive each other as a burden. Of course we would not expect such an interaction to continue very long on a voluntary basis. Although other combinations are possible, it is not my intention here to review all of them. The above examples were cited as illustrations.

I would venture the opinion that in our interactions with others we try to be an asset in all spheres of our activities. We are an asset to our society if we contribute to the material and emotional well-being of our fellow society members. This means being a productive member of society and psychologically supportive to as many people as possible for as long as possible.

THE IMPACT OF DISEASE ON THE INDIVIDUAL

We view the diseased state as a maladjustment between the individual and the environment. This maladjustment causes a perception of "absence of ease" at the conscious level. If this so-called "absence of ease" reaches significant proportions, the individual is considered ill. A sick person cannot help but become a burden to others, either psychologically, financially, or physically, or any combination thereof. Thus the quality of life of the diseased person is affected and so is the life of those around him or her.

In order to evaluate the impact of a disease on an individual, we need standards, a point of reference against which our measurements can be made. Given human variability, universal standards are difficult to find. This issue was addressed by Carl Cohen (1985) who concluded that there are some generalized and some individualized features that affect the quality of life. Some of the generalized features add to the quality of life while others detract from it. The positive, additive features include intelligence, mobility, physical stamina, and length of life. Negative features include confinement to bed or to an institution, mental instability, fear, and intense or chronic pain. Individualized features consist of life experiences that fulfill us or frustrate us in conducting our life.

Cohen proposes the recognition of what he calls a "life plan." He argues that each of us lives our lives with some degree of coherence. We all have goals and purposes that distinguish us from others. In life we identify ourselves with several roles, such as family and professional roles, and we identify ourselves with causes and principles which we are willing to defend. While the life plan of one person might be judged by others as either worthy or frivolous, rational or irrational, nevertheless the life plan of the individual should serve as the standard against which we can measure the degree of loss in the quality of his or her life.

Key areas of quality of life that were of concern to patients were: interpersonal relations (marriage, family, friends); sexual adjustment; work function; leisure activities; and physical and emotional symptoms, e.g., pain, anxiety, sadness (Cohen-Cole 1986).

Several methods have been introduced to measure the extent of functional impairment. Some of these are specific for certain kinds of disabilities while others measure general impairment.

Specific evaluations include the Physical Status Scale of the American Society of Anesthesiologists, the Apgar Score for evaluating newborns for functional impairment, the New York Heart Association criteria for functional impairment in heart disease, the American Rheumatism Association

(ARA) functional scale, the Iowa Hip Score for evaluating hip disabilities, the Visick Classification for evaluating post-gastrectomy patients, the Karnofsky Index for assessing the effectiveness of cancer treatment, the Adaptive Balance Profile to measure the psychological outcomes of illness, and the Psychosocial Adjustment to Illness Scale to measure the psychosocial outcomes of illness.

The following methods have been introduced to measure the general impact of a diseased state: the Barthel Index, the PULSES Profile, the Sickness Impact Profile, the Northingham Health Profile (NHP) and Spitzer's QL-Index.

Our purpose here is to provide an overall orientation and not to appraise the different methods. The interested reader is referred to texts on rehabilitation. Several references can be found in an article by O'Young, McPeek and Mosteller (1985).

The quantification and thus measurement of disabilities can be of use in health policy planning where it can help in resource allocation and in evaluating the impact of the disease on a population. Additional uses include direct clinical application where such measurement can assist in clinical decision making by (1) determining the impact of the disease on the individual physically as well as psychologically, and (2) by assessing the rate of recovery or the rate of progression of a disease and thus measuring the effectiveness of treatment.

THE IMPACT OF ILLNESS ON "SIGNIFICANT OTHERS"

All the measures discussed earlier deal with the diseased person. The scales and measurements were designed to answer the questions, "What does the disease mean for society?" and "What does the disease mean to the affected person?" Our current dynamic view of health and disease and of interpersonal relations implies that the disease of a person has consequences not only for the affected person but also for those who interact with him or her.

It is rather curious that we do not have a measure for the burden a diseased person presents for those caring for him. To say it another way, How much burden is placed on those who care for a diseased person? How much does a caregiver contribute to the recovery of a sick person? How much is required from a caregiver to be an effective helper? These are related questions and we have no answer to any of them. We know well that the illness of a family member can represent a physical burden — for instance, the sick person has to be assisted with personal hygiene or feeding—as well as a financial and psychological burden. It is my feeling that in cases not requiring extensive institutional care, the burden of the disease is greater on those who feel responsible for the patient than it is on society. Yet we have no measure for this large contribution to the welfare of the sick.

Families who have a child with muscular dystrophy spend many hours in caring for the child, in providing transportation for him to school and to medical appointments, spending effort and money in adapting their house to the child's needs. They sacrifice vacations because the special care required by the child depletes their financial resources. The time they would have available for recreation and for intimacies is severely curtailed, thus the quality of the care other children receive might be lessened. There is also a large amount of psychological distress associated with the care of a sick family member, especially if it is a young person.

It would be one-sided to speak only of the burden a sick person represents. In the care of the sick we find a manifestation of humankind very different from the brute force and heartless exploitation we so often witness in the economic and political arena. Witnessing suffering seems to keep the humanitarian spirit alive. Thus our sick indirectly contribute to society by reminding us of our vulnerability and thus making us more compassionate.

The ill are also often a source of inspiration. We have all had the occasion to marvel at the achievements of the handicapped, be uplifted by their spirit and touched by their enthusiasm for life. We have no measurements for these values, yet we should. Similarly, we are not likely to find a measure, at least not in dollars and cents, for an understanding hug, for a sympathetic ear, or for a loving smile. What is the value of a smile that is made to appear on a sad face? How can we measure tears that have been wiped off?

We do not even have a good measure of the economic value of the lives saved by health professionals. We only have measurements for the amount of money the treatment requires and for the production lost because of the absence of the patients from work.

As for the psychological effects of the health care workers in providing encouragement, giving reassurance, relieving anxiety, keeping hope alive, and thus making life's struggles more bearable, we do not even have an approximation.

The cost of health care is scrutinized repeatedly by insurance companies and government agencies. These studies, however, do not take into account many of the benefits that society receives from the infirm and do not count contributions from family members, health care workers, and others who provide psychological help along with their more palpable contribution.

As was pointed out by Cassell (1982) "No person exists without others. This is doubly true for the sick person who depends on others for his or her daily existence. It is in relationships with others that the full range of human emotions finds expression." Do we wish to deny the value of emotions? We have seen the prominent role emotion is given in promotional campaigns and in personal improvement programs. Because thus far economic measurements have been unable to penetrate the realms of interpersonal relations, the psychological benefits that the patient receives from others remain uncounted, while the importance of emotional factors in recovery is acknowledged. We give theoretical recognition to the importance of treating the whole person by paying attention to both body and mind, but recognize only that part of the contribution by the caregivers which concerns the body. Simply because the psychological impact is difficult to measure, we do not account for the *total* care accorded to the patient. Thus much of our health statistics concerned with cost-benefit calculations of health care are grossly inadequate.

THE IMPACT OF ILLNESS
ON HEALTH CARE PERSONNEL

A special kind of interaction takes place between the patient and health care professionals. The health care providers cannot help but be affected by the sufferings and triumphs of their patients. In chronic illnesses, such as muscular dystrophy, the triumphs become fewer and the setbacks more numerous as time goes on.

The master clinician, Sir William Osler, was well aware of this problem and recommended compassion, provision of the best possible care, and the cultivation of a certain degree of emotional indifference. He just felt that uncontrolled emotions would interfere with clinical judgement and thus would compromise the care of the patient. According to Osler (1953) ". . . in the physician or surgeon no quality takes rank with imperturbability . . . coolness and presence of mind under all circumstances . . . . Keen sensibility is doubtless a virtue of high order, when it does not interfere with steadiness of hand or coolness of nerve." His advice: "Cultivate, then, gentlemen, such a judicious measure of obtuseness as will enable you to meet the exigencies of practice with firmness and courage, without, at the same time, hardening 'The human heart by which we live.' "

RESPONDING TO THE TOTAL NEEDS
OF THE PATIENT

Recently several attempts have been made to enlarge the physician's armamentarium in responding to the needs of the whole patient. Beside concentrating on the physical manifestation of illness, attention is given to the emotional state of the patient. This expanded view has not only theoretical importance but has practical value as well. It has been shown that patients' adherence to medical regimens and the physical outcome of treatment are positively influenced by the physician's ability to help the patient cope with his or her emotions (DiMatteo and Friedman 1982).

An unsatisfactory patient-physician relationship can result in a resentful or angry patient. This is clearly counterproductive in both the therapeutic and financial sense. Angry patients can lash out at the physician, can criticize support staff, might change doctors, can complain to patient care representatives, or file a lawsuit (Lazare 1987). The importance of paying attention to more than the obvious physical findings at hand is underscored by a recent statistical survey which demonstrated that more than half of patients changed doctors because they were dissatisfied with their doctor's attitude (*Physician's Management*, April 1987). The importance of good interpersonal relationships was likewise stressed by a business-oriented article. The author advises doctors to rate themselves on the "four As" which are believed to be important for a successful practitioner: Accessibility, Affability, Availability and Affordability. Here affability refers to good patient-doctor relationship (Brooten, Jr. 1987).

It has been proposed that although patients experience many complex emotions, there are three basic types of emotional reactions that can cause difficulty for the physician. These are anger, fear, and sadness (Ekman 1975).

A guide was prepared by Cohen-Cole and Bird (1986) for physicians to help patients cope with their emotions. They stress the importance of both verbal and nonverbal communication. Discussing verbal intervention, they focus on five attitudes that the physician should attempt to communicate to the patients: empathy, legitimation, support, partnership, and respect. They add, however, that caring can be communicated most effectively through nonverbal behaviors such as direct eye contact, a foreward lean indicating interest, appropriate physical distance, head nodding, and open posture.

Complicating factors in patient-doctor interaction can stem from our unique personhood and from situational circumstances. A counterthera-peutic situation can be created by the following settings: (1) the dependent, burdensome position of the patient providing a fertile ground for the development of certain personality characteristics that can lead to clashes with caregivers; (2) the presence of certain characteristics in the caregivers that are in conflict with some of the patient's characteristics; and (3) situational difficulties.

Patient characteristics that are liable to lead to problems in patient-caregiver relationships can be grouped into two categories: those for which the patient is thought to be responsible because they are under the patient's control, and those for which the patient is not thought to be responsible. According to Levinson (1985) patients with characteristics for which they are held responsible are described as:

- Emotional/Unreasonable/Hysterical;
- Highly dependent;
- Passive aggressive;
- Controlling/Independent;
- Ingratiating/Flattering/Seducing;
- Manipulative/Deceitful;
- Uncooperative/Undisciplined;
- Medical system abusers;
- Demanding/Complaining;
- Having low pain tolerance;
- Self-destructive (substance abuser/smoker/suicidal);
- Health faddist/Know-it-all.

Characteristics of patients for which they are not held liable but can lead to difficult patient-caregiver relationships include:

- Ignorance/Low Intelligence/Mental retardation;
- Psychosis;
- Terminal illness;
- Undiagnosable condition;
- Victims of tragic life circumstances.

Characteristics of physicians that are liable to lead to conflict with certain patient's characteristics were likewise listed by Levinson (1985). It is noteworthy that several of these are considered virtues by general societal standards:

- Scientific/Objective/Reasonable;
- Unemotional;
- Responsible/Conscientious;
- Perfectionist;

- Seeking mastery and control;
- Dependent/Need to be needed;
- Overly cautious/Afraid of harming;
- Seeking status among peers and community;
- Idealistic/Altruistic/Self-sacrificing;
- Self-reliant/Disciplined;
- Rescuing/Heroic;
- Highly ethical;
- Needing personal time for family and recreation.

Situational difficulties can interfere with orderly patient-caregiver relationships. Examples of these are time pressure, excessive paperwork, administrative overcontrol, the patient's inability to afford necessary care, inadequate physical environment (e.g., "the hustle and bustle" of a large urban hospital), intimidating high-tech equipment, and patients' embarrassment at having their bodies exposed and probed by strangers.

To reduce the shame and humiliation of a medical encounter Lazare (1987) provides us with the following recommendations:

- Create an environment that is as human and welcoming as possible;
- See patients with minimum delay;
- Address patients with their proper titles and surnames; and
- Protect the privacy of the patients' bodies, verbal disclosures, and records.

EPILOGUE

Increasingly, in our age of advancing mechanization, cost-containment and accountability, people are becoming statistics, and human interactions are regarded as services or encounters. In order to save ourselves from complete dehumanization, emphasis should be placed on two human characteristics: individuality and the necessity of interaction.

Individual uniqueness demands flexibility in our approach to fellow human beings. It demands respect for differences in appearance and for diversity in desire, opinion, action, and reaction. Individuals afflicted with the same disease tolerate it differently. The same medicine is metabolized differently in different individuals and the dosage that might be therapeutic in one could prove to be toxic in another. Exposure to infectious agents under identical conditions causes illness in some while others remain healthy. And the phenomenon of different people witnessing the same event and reaching differing conclusions forms the stuff of party politics.

Interaction with others is a necessity, both in health and in disease. Thus the understanding of the patient-caregiver relationship requires close attention to interactional dynamics. The approach proposed here is based on value-perception, whereby others are perceived as assets, burdens, or incidentals. It was pointed out that our interactions take place in at least three spheres: the physical, the psychological, and the economic, and that in each sphere we can perceive assets and burdens. This approach revealed that our measurements regarding the provision of health care measure cost-benefit effects in the economic and physical spheres, while similar interactions in the psychological sphere remain largely uncounted.

I prefer to call the type of analysis applied here, which is centered on the individual, recognizing his uniqueness and seeing him in constant interaction with his environment, as *contextual individualism*.

At one time the introduction of computers was regarded as a possible dehumanizing influence and a tool of mass regimentation. I propose that if we collectively step forward, the new generation of computers with their greatly increased storage and calculating capacity can become our allies. They are able to handle the increased amount of information that a consideration of individual variability and environmental peculiarity would demand. Instead of being classified into a few categories, with the help of the "super-computers" our individuality, in the realm of numbers, can receive increasing recognition.

The uniqueness of the individual and the complexity of environments dictates that our approach to patients with muscular dystrophy, as well as other diseases, should be greatly individualized. We should recognize each patient's individual assets, be cognizant of his or her individual liabilities, and incorporate this knowledge into the treatment plan. Let us hope that, until the day when a cure will finally appear on the horizon, a treatment plan based on *contextual individualism* will result in improved quality of life for patients and their families.

REFERENCES

Brooten, K. E. Jr. 1987. "Establishing Effective Patient Relationships." *Physician's Management* (May):203-237.

Cassell, E. J. 1982. "The Nature of Suffering and the Goals of Medicine." *New England Journal of Medicine* 306(11): 639-645.

Cohen, C. 1985. "Psychosocial Reflections on the Impact of Coronary Artery Surgery on Patients' Quality of Life." *Quality of Life and Cardiovascular Care* (May/June):209-214.

Cohen-Cole, S. A. 1985. "Interviewing the Cardiac Patient I: A Practical Guide for Assessing Quality of Life." *Quality of Life and Cardiovascular Care* (November/December):7-12.

Cohen-Cole, S. A. and J. Bird. 1986. "Interviewing the Cardiac Patient II: A Practical Guide for Helping Patients Cope with Their Emotions." *Quality of Life and Cardiovascular Care* (January/February):53-65.

DiMatteo, R. and H. Friedman. 1982. "Patient Cooperation with Treatment." In R. DiMatteo and H. Friedman, eds. *Social Psychology and Medicine*. Cambridge, MA: Oelgeschlager, Gunn and Hain, pp. 35-38.

"Doctor-Patient Relations Key in Patient Retention." April, 1987. *Physician's Management*, p. 15.

Ekman, P. 1975. "Unmasking the Face: A Guide to Recognizing Emotions from Facial Clues." Englewood Cliffs, NJ: Prentice Hall.

Jung, C. G. 1965. "The Soul and Death." In H. Feifel, ed. *The Meaning of Death*. New York: McGraw-Hill, pp. 3-15.

Lazare, A. Cited in *Medical World News*, December 28, 1987, p. 34.

Levinson, D. 1985. "Counter-Therapeutic Reactions to Patients." *Physician and Patient* (June):18-22.

Osler, W. 1953. *Aequanimitas*. Third Edition. New York: Blakiston.

O'Young, J., B. McPeek, and F. Mosteller. 1985. "The Clinician's Role in Developing Measures for Quality of Life in Cardiovascular Disease." *Quality of Life and Cardiovascular Care* (July/August):290-296.

Emotional Stress
and Multiple Sclerosis

Bruce L. Danto

Many people who have professional medical contact with patients suffering from multiple sclerosis have observed that these are people who have severe emotional problems. Of course, one might be able to make this observation about any person who suffers from a disease that tends to be chronic and grossly debilitating. Certain differences can be noted among those suffering from multiple sclerosis with respect to their personality types and their way of dealing with emotional conflict. Therefore, it is the purpose of this essay to attempt to highlight one part of the emotional aspect of this disease, namely, any relationship that may exist between emotional stress and the onset of the disease. Additionally, a review of the literature pertinent to this area of investigation is summarized along with the presentation of five cases which, it is hoped, will serve to illustrate the nature of such a relationship.

LITERATURE REVIEW

Most research relating psychological factors to onset of multiple sclerosis was done in the 1940s and 1950s. In an early account of two cases published by Voss (1943), it was stated that there might be some relationship between severe emotional trauma and the onset of multiple sclerosis. The title of the article was misleading because it implied that a specific emotional trauma precipitated the development of multiple sclerosis, but an examination of the two cases showed that the symptoms had already been present for years. In reality, they were chronic multiple sclerotic patients with severe exacerbations resulting from the acute emotional trauma of air raid bombings.

Bruce L. Danto, MD, is affiliated with the Neuromuscular Clinic, Mount Sinai Hospital and Medical Center, New York, NY 10029.

Other investigators such as Borberg and Zahle (1946) have proposed the existence of a psychological predisposition or premorbid personality. Further, they suspected that pathogenic noxae have the power to set in motion a chain reaction of psychiatric manifestations of the preexisting factors. Such investigators feel that one measure of the relevancy of their hypothesis is the fact that mental changes occur during the first three years of the onset of the disease. Of all the varied types of psychiatric manifestations, the two most prominent are euphoria and dementia. Cited as preexisting factors are tendencies toward hypochondria, self-directed interests, and infantilism.

Langworthy (1948, 1950) discussed the frequency with which patients are seen and diagnosed as having conversion hysteria, only later to be proven to have multiple sclerosis after the signs of organic brain disease appear. He postulated that many such persons show premorbid personality characteristics seen in conversion hysteria. These people are emotionally immature and may not have reached even an adolescent stage of personality development. He recorded their histories of inadequacy in dealing with sexual problems and anxieties over sex. He felt they convert anxiety into physical symptoms. Such persons are passive-dependent people who are resentful of domineering, aggressive persons. Langworthy felt that female patients are frequently tied to their mothers and tend to marry weak, passive men, suffering symptoms of conversion when the men become more aggressive and domineering. He attributed the euphoria of the multiple sclerosis person to anxiety which has been converted. Although his ideas were speculative, he suspected that emotional disturbances might induce cerebral vascular spasm producing organic changes which in turn lead to the lesions associated with the disease.

In his discussion he reported a case of a young man who presented with symptoms two days after he had completed a course of clinical neurology. The patient had achieved remission following psychotherapy. Unmentioned, however, was the prospect that his remission might represent a cyclical one characteristic of the disease. Langworthy felt that psychotherapy is particularly important during periods of emotional turmoil and offers promise in averting a worsening of patients' organic symptoms because of the possible vaso-motor reflexes. In some cases he found evidence of worsening symptoms associated with increased turmoil and stress in the patient's relationships with other people.

Grinker, Haur, and Robbins (1950) studied 46 patients with multiple sclerosis and found histories of mothers whom the patients could never reach emotionally and fathers who were often alcoholic, sadistic, and deserted their families. Such families were not close and later emotional attachments of such persons were superficial at best. Their sexual interests were minimal and became diminished as the disease progressed. Of interest was the frequency of major changes in the life situation as a precipitating factor for the development of overt neurologic symptoms. Such changes included the death of loved ones, desertion, and an anxiety-producing addition of responsibilities. Remissions were commensurate with ameliorations of these stresses. Fundamentally, their patients demonstrated an excessive need for love and affection which had not been gratified in childhood. These qualities constitute Grinker's concept of the premorbid personality of the multiple sclerotic patient who attempts to meet these needs by developing a "happy-go-lucky" personality. He displays a need to please and receive approval, showing an outward calm but experiencing an inner tension.

Grinker et al. suspected a pathophysiologic etiology of multiple sclerosis in terms of defects in the development of myelinization of human infants during the first two years of life. They postulated that these patients are indeed quite infantile and might have a greater constitutional need for external supplies of unknown enzymes and lipids. Further, they wondered about a disruption of the biochemical process in terms of an imbalance induced by stress such as physical or even significant emotional deprivation. Such stress was reflected in the emotional developmental histories of the people studied. They postulated that demyelinization could occur subsequently so that psychologically as well as neurologically they become the infants they emotionally wanted to be. Such a concept had been suspected earlier by Hollos and Ferenczi (1925), who felt that psychic disorders in "demential paralytica" are regressions to earlier levels of neurologic development.

Pratt (1951) took issue with Grinker et al., contending that his comparison of 100 multiple sclerosis patients versus 100 control cases failed to demonstrate the "happy-go-lucky" type of premorbid personality. Further, albeit there was no statistical significance between the multiple sclerosis and control group, Pratt did feel that there were some cases in which emotional antecedents could be established to show an associated or subsequent onset of multiple sclerosis.

Brickner and Simons (1950) studied 50 patients with multiple sclerosis and reported a large number of cases in which emotional stress existed in relation to the onset of the condition. They felt that one could speculate on the role of stress as a precipitant or arbiter of regression. Notwithstanding their intuitive feelings, they felt the ultimate proof would lie in giving specific emotional shocks to patients with known multiple sclerosis by way of some experimental design. Furthermore, they discussed instances when emotional factors did not induce an exacerbation of symptoms because the factor might be potent at one time and not at another. They were firm in their suspicion that emotional stress might provoke the disease or its attacks even though not causing it. Cases were clearer when the interval was short between the time of stress and the onset of pathologic neurologic process and conversely more suspect when one could record a long interval of time. In long interval cases, conditions of anorexia and gastrointestinal symptoms ensued. They speculated that the latter symptoms might have been transient somatic expressions in the interim between stress and the appearance of the neurologic manifestations. The latter situation is seen in case No. 2 reported below.

Harrower and Kraus (1951) proposed that although they failed to find evidence of a stereotypical picture of a presumptive multiple sclerotic personality, there were findings of note on various psychometric tests conducted on such patients. The test data showed characteristics such as an overemphasis of dependency needs, absolute absence of body-centered anxiety, a minimum of inner conflict, and an attitude of resignation. They displayed a type of unrealistic "rose-colored-glasses" approach to life. The incidence of such traits in multiple sclerosis patients was infinitely higher than in the control group involved in their study. However, there were a few patients who individually showed deviation from the characteristics recorded as an overall group pattern.

Harrower (1954) found that psychological characteristics could not be considered as predisposing a person to multiple sclerosis, since when certain conditions were varied, they showed different responses on psychological tests. This was demonstrated in the area of dependency needs. When such needs were altered, the patients were encouraged to develop more independence. However, the program was carried out in a highly protective type of rehabilitation setting, one in which dependency might be disguised in a patient's adjustment because of external control over stress. Independence in this type of milieu might be reflected on a more superficial level and not be quite as apparent when looking at the patient in his own natural milieu.

Baldwin (1952) investigated a number of psychological aspects in the study of 34 women who were suffering from multiple sclerosis. She compared them with a control group of 34 normal women. The two groups were matched closely as to educational background, marital status, age, maternity status, I.Q. level and cultural background. Her data showed that multiple sclerosis patients present themselves as well-adjusted. They utilized denial and rationalization to smooth over events which should have elicited an affect more appropriate to the traumatic situation. Repression was the defense utilized by the multiple sclerosis patient more often than by the controls. The controls showed more self-awareness of feelings than multiple sclerosis patients. The multiple sclerosis patients used denial to defend against guilt feelings and anxiety-arousing wishes much in the same way that has been seen in cases of hysteria. Like the hysterical personality, the multiple sclerosis patient was suggestible and tended to use the organic condition for secondary gain.

To summarize the research investigations of this problem, it has been frequently found and/or suspected that the multiple sclerosis patient has a passive-dependent type of premorbid personality, one easily upset by emotional stress or trauma. Such patients tend to utilize repression and denial as ego-defenses to cope with anxiety. They superficially present themselves as "happy-go-lucky" people whose suffering is completely internalized.

CASE ILLUSTRATIONS

These cases were selected from ones seen at the Wayne State University, College of Medicine, Multiple Sclerosis Clinic. These patients were interviewed over a period of two weeks. One of the patients was hospitalized at the time of the interviews. The case reports do not contain diagnostic, clinical and laboratory data since they had all been evaluated previously and their diagnosis was established prior to the interview.

Case No. 1

The patient is a 26-year-old, white, single male. The onset of his neurologic problems was dated to September, 1962, two weeks following his fiancee's termination of their engagement. They had been engaged for three months after a courtship of over a year. He had met her while she was still in high school. Since he had graduated they decided to postpone an engagement until she completed her high school education. Subsequent to their engagement, she fell in love with an old childhood sweetheart and it was for this reason that she terminated the engagement and later married the other man.

The onset of his neurologic problem was marked by symptoms of easy fatigability, light-headedness relieved by sitting down, and blurred vision. Three months later, diplopia occurred. He had some early signs of bladder and bowel incontinence and paresthesias on the left side of his body excluding his face at that time.

In November, 1962, following hospitalization, he was diagnosed by a neurologist as having multiple sclerosis, but he was not informed of his diagnosis until May, 1963. In December, 1962, the patient was told by his former fiancee that she was pregnant. She implied that he was the father, but that she had delayed telling him this. Subsequently, she went to another state to deliver her child, which she later placed out for adoption. She returned home in April, 1963, one month prior to the patient's being informed of his diagnosis. She was married six months later.

From the time the patient was informed of his diagnosis, he underwent a progressive deterioration. In late September, 1963, prior to another hospitalization, he became unable to walk. He became more incapacitated with bowel and bladder incontinence and paresthesias. There was an exacerbation of his condition in September, 1963, a date one year following the time when his fiancee terminated their engagement.

With respect to his earlier history, his health prior to the onset of multiple sclerosis had been good. The medical history consisted of a torn medical meniscus of his left knee as a result of a football injury in the 12th grade of high school and an episode of infectious mononucleosis in the 7th grade. He was described by himself and his family as being a somewhat "happy-go-lucky" type of person prior to the onset of his immediate illness. He was a shy young man, despite the fact that he had made a varsity letter in football while in high school. The patient likened himself to his father, whom he described as a very passive type of man, dominated by the patient's mother, whom he considered as the more assertive of the two parents. Since the onset of his illness he felt he had tried at times to take his feelings out on his parents, to express his resentment about having multiple sclerosis. At times, he blamed his parents. As a result, he had felt a great deal of guilt and was upset by the fact that his father never responded to his attacks. It was always his mother who "cuts me down to size."

The patient was employed as a truck driver following graduation from high school. He was the second of three children, the oldest of whom is a 31-year-old, married and financially successful sister. A 23-year-old, single brother has had frequent contacts with the police because of reckless driving and an accumulation of traffic violations associated with alcoholic intoxication.

With respect to his sexual adjustment, it should be indicated that his fiancee was his first sexual experience and she was described as a very attractive blond who was attracted to the patient primarily because of his good looks and the fact that he was a "big man" on the football team.

Case No. 2

The patient is a 64-year-old, white, single female. The onset of her multiple sclerosis was dated to February, 1959, with the appearance of blurred vision and almost complete blindness of her right eye.

Her mother died in January, 1948, at age 81, of heart disease, and her father died of myocarditis with heart block in April, 1958, at age 84. The patient had cared for her parents for most of her life prior to their death. Subsequent to her mother's death, the patient, who had had an excellent health history without any significant problems, began to complain of epigastric pain of an intermittent, dull aching nature, as well as insomnia, a symptom which still persists. Significantly, her father had a chronic history of intestinal symptoms associated with adhesions of the intestines. He also had a mucous colitis. As her parents had been considerably weakened from the effects of old age and their chronic medical conditions, her financial support was necessary.

Prior to her parents' deaths, the patient had worked as a power machine operator in a pants factory and had been self-sufficient and able to support her parents. Her health had been good except for two D and C's because of menorrhagia in 1951. Regarding her employment, she said, "I always worried about being in the way, but I paid my bills." In 1957, the plant where she had been employed for 16 years moved and it was necessary for her to find a new job. At the new place of employment, she was unable to maintain her production as in the past and thereafter went from job to job. While under much financial pressure, her physical symptoms intensified. It was in 1959 that the onset of her multiple sclerosis was marked by the development of blurred vision and complete blindness of the right eye.

Following her father's death in 1958, she went to live with her brother and sister-in-law. The brother is her only sibling and is 68 years old. The patient was not too welcome in her brother's home, but did remain there until her sister-in-law, who is diabetic and hypertensive, felt she could no longer care for the patient. One incident that reflects the feelings of the brother and sister-in-law regarding their care of the patient concerned the events of her only proposal of marriage. At age 50, she dated a man for 12 months until 1956. Despite encouragement on the part of her brother to marry the man, she was unable to tolerate his sexual advances. She broke off with him, but he kept calling and her brother and sister-in-law kept pressuring her to marry him. She became distressed about the situation because she felt that they were trying to get rid of her. She felt a sense of loss because most of her life had been devoted to taking care of her parents and she consciously felt she did not miss going out with men.

Since June, 1963, the patient has been residing in a convalescent home, an arrangement about which she is most unhappy. She has become depressed and upset about not being able to be at home with her brother. She complains of musculoskeletal pain, which has become worse, particularly since she has been upset over her new living arrangements.

Additional historical background includes the fact that she had a 9th grade education, quitting school in order to go to work to contribute support to the family. It was at this time that she obtained employment as a special machine operator at a pants manufacturing company.

In March, 1961, it was felt that the patient might be suffering from conversion hysteria. She was admitted to the psychiatric service of a local hospital as she was depressed, cried constantly, and refused to walk despite the absence of an organic basis for this symptom.

With reference to her feelings about having multiple sclerosis, her primary thought has been, "I'm happy my parents did not have to see me this way. I was always happy to do things for others." The patient gives the appearance of being a somewhat mouse-like, thin woman who has "shriveled up." She is very meek and passive and shows much underlying depression despite her superficial light-heartedness.

Case No. 3

The patient is a 52-year-old, white, married male. The onset of his multiple sclerosis was dated to 1958, the time he learned that it would be necessary to sell his home because of financial problems. The onset was marked by blurred vision and problems of coordination. He had noticed his vision was not as "keen as it used to be." As he became intensely depressed over having had to sell the house he stopped working as a pattern maker. He was further upset over criticism by his wife and two daughters regarding his problems of coordination. In the latter regard he said, "I suffer a lot emotionally because I can't stand criticism. That really hurts; I would welcome a definite end of my life. No use wishing because no one dies of multiple sclerosis, just the effects of multiple sclerosis. I don't want sympathy, but my oldest daughter is as mean as hell and expects too much!"

With reference to his family history, he indicated that his mother had died of a heart attack in 1950. His father had died in 1959 of multiple ailments, involving diabetes associated with urinary incontinence, ulcerations of the legs, and peripheral vascular insufficiency. His father had had great difficulty in walking. He was an alcoholic and the patient said, "He was the meanest god-damned person in the world. I would see my mother crying from his abuse, such as hitting her and us kids. There were times when I was even afraid to come into the house when I was a kid. Mother loved the kids. She loved the boys. She was good. She was the best mother, but a god-damned poor wife, just like my wife.'' Of interest is the fact that frequently throughout the interview he would refer to his wife as ''my mother'' and then would seem to catch himself and correct the word to ''wife.''

The patient had purchased a house, which he deeply loved, in early 1958. It was purchased against the protest and constant criticism of his wife and two daughters. He said, ''It made me heartsick when I had to sell it. I cried inside. I'm just like a utility man, I have no say in my house. I used to try to get my way and was accused of always getting my way. They (referring to his wife and two daughters) accused me of being God almighty, like my father. Since I've gotten multiple sclerosis, I'm totally defenseless and get cut off easily.'' The patient described himself as a ''worry bird'' type of person. His wife would refer to their home as ''your house.''

She showed much fear in regard to becoming pregnant and expected the patient to use prophylactics. They have not had sexual relations for the past three years. In this regard, he said, ''I used to be pretty sexy, once or twice per week.'' He felt that he had become impotent as a result of a lack of encouragement from his wife.

The patient's older brother was sickly and was described by the patient as being a ''hypochondriac.'' There is an unmarried 28-year-old daughter who treats this brother as the patient's two daughters treat him. In his childhood, the brother apparently was ''babied'' a great deal. Their mother was prone to ''baby her boys.'' The brother was discharged from the Army with a diagnosis of psychoneurosis.

The patient was in the Navy during World War II and had undertaken specialized training in electronics, but he had failed his third advanced electrician school placement. He was a high school graduate and had been interested in electronics for many years, but despite this, he worked as a pattern maker.

Case No. 4

The patient is a 42-year-old, white, married female. The onset of her multiple sclerosis was dated to 1960 at the time her husband was complaining of chest pain and palpitations. Although his symptoms later proved to be due to cardiac anxiety, she was concerned that her husband had organic heart disease. An associated worry was his inability to obtain life insurance because of this diagnosis. Prior to the definite diagnosis that was eventually made, she developed central visual blindness in the right eye. At this same time, her daughter sustained severe burns and the patient's brother was trapped in a hot rod race car that caught fire. The events of the latter accident were witnessed by the patient with much anxiety despite the fact that the brother was uninjured. Coincident to the above stresses, the patient's other daughter almost drowned in a wading pool. Two years later, she was further upset when she was notified by the State that the home that she and her husband had built themselves had been condemned for purposes of an expressway project.

In 1956, the patient and her husband had opened a small business dealing in the repair and sale of motorcycles. In reference to those early years of business struggles, she said, "We practically starved for the first three or four years."

The patient's parents were described by her as being "Quiet, church-going, nondrinking people who owned their own farm. Mother made our clothes and would go without shoes to give us some. They're as poor as church mice." In 1963, her mother fell down the steps, receiving a cerebral concussion and later developing a toxemic type of hypertensive reaction, a condition about which the patient was most concerned.

The patient has two brothers and one sister and is number three in ordinal position. Her sister currently does all the patient's shopping; she and the patient have always been very close. In regard to their relationship, the patient said, "We're not sisters, we are the best of friends. She comes over and washes my hair and takes care of my kids." The patient's siblings are in good health and all of the children were born at home except for the fourth child, the one which followed the patient.

Regarding her husband she commented, "He is good to me. I get anything within his power to get for me." Of herself she said, "I was always lazy, my sister always took to work easier than I did. I had to take care of two kids and help my husband at the store and it was rough. Until we took on the business I took things in my stride, but when we took on the business I went the opposite way. When he took sick, I worried, 'How am I going to run the shop and care for the kids if anything happens to him?' He couldn't get a job or insurance or anything and I was very upset."

The patient is a high school graduate, but felt "dumb" in school compared to her peers who had benefit of private Catholic schooling. Her physical health as a child, with the exception of diptheria at nine years of age, was excellent. The mother had told her that one of her brothers died of diptheria, but the patient was more fortunate and recovered after having been bedridden for a period of two weeks.

With reference to her attitudes and feelings about sex, she said, "I've never been very sexy and he has never pushed himself on me. My husband has been understanding. We have never had much to do with one another since March, 1963. I've only achieved orgasm a few times since we have been married. I was afraid, it hurt so bad. I'm chicken."

In describing her parents she said that her mother was the most assertive of the two and was responsible for the punishment of the children and making the important decisions.

The patient recalls one childhood nightmare of having been chased by a bulldog who wanted to bite her.

Case No. 5

The patient is a 42-year-old, white, married male who is currently subsisting on Social Security. The onset of his condition was dated to summer, 1958, at which time, for unexplained reasons, he became unhappy about having to do "close work" on his job. Precision work on his hand-operated screw machine, which required measurements in terms of tenths, was upsetting to him. He performed his work at an aircraft plant. His depression over his unexplained concern about the close work intensified. In 1960, without being urged by anyone, he entered treatment with a psychiatrist who saw him for 20 appointments over a six-month period. As he felt he was not getting relief from his depression or achieving understanding of his problem, he terminated treatment. In reference to this, the patient said, "I wanted him to find out what was wrong with me." Subsequently, he began to miss days of work. In early January, 1962, he began to complain of left-sided paresthesias, weakness of his left leg, ataxia and decreased vision without blurring or diplopia. His family doctor recommended and arranged for the patient's admission to a local hospital, where a diagnosis of multiple sclerosis was made. He was discharged shortly after, and at this time he quit his job. He began to complain of sexual impotence. Since that particular time he has been living on Social Security.

Family history revealed that he has one sibling, a brother 10 years younger. He and the patient have not seen one another for three years as the brother lives out of the state. The brother is an electronic engineer. Both of the patient's parents are living in Arizona and are in good health, as is the patient's brother. His father was a tailor at a department store and the patient described him as always being too busy to see the patient when he was a child. Discipline was performed by the mother and it was always she who spanked, but only rarely. The father was a nondrinker and is now 82 years of age. The mother is about 76 years of age. The patient revealed that his mother was the more assertive of the two and seemed to run the house and make the major decisions as regards her children.

The patient's physical health history was excellent prior to the onset of his multiple sclerosis, except for pneumonia at 8 years of age. He described himself as being a "happy-go-lucky" type of person who "always wanted to forget anything painful. I think of something else which is more pleasant."

He attended school until 11A and subsequently quit to go into the service, but was rejected because of a right inguinal hernia. Instead of returning to school, he obtained employment as a mill machine operator in 1943. He was always shy about dating girls prior to his marriage. He married at the age of 26 without experience prior to marriage. Subsequent to marriage they had intercourse once a week. However, because of his impotence, he has been unable to have intercourse since June, 1962. His wife has accepted his impotence. They had never had an affectionate type of relationship and he felt that his wife was the more assertive in regard to running the house, raising the children and making the major decisions.

The patient has thought about committing suicide, but without definite fantasies. In regard to the latter, he said, "There wouldn't be blood involved though. I saw a guy shot and blown up while hunting once. When I think of it, I stop and think of something else more pleasant." He gave much evidence of being preoccupied with wanting to forget unpleasant things. He covered up unpleasant thoughts by repression and a euphoria which has been persistant since the diagnosis of multiple sclerosis was made. It was difficult to see evidence of depression because of his euphoria.

Since his discharge from the hospital he has complained of a constant claustrophobia, which he would experience in church, in the examining room when he comes to clinic for check-ups, and even at the time this particular interview was conducted. He said, "I can't stand being boxed in." Of speculative significance is the fact that the most common type of punishment the patient received as a child was being kept in the house and in his room by his mother.

DISCUSSION

The cases reported in the above section all illustrate the presence of emotional stress preceeding the onset of multiple sclerosis. The cases do show some variation in that in Nos. 1 and 3, there was a sudden onset following an acute, emotionally traumatic situation. In case No. 2, there is a less exact or less well-defined relationship between the various emotional stresses on the patient – the parents' deaths, the loss of her job – and the onset of her multiple sclerosis. This case also illustrates the problem of a differential diagnosis between multiple sclerosis and hysteria, as was commented on in the introduction of this paper. Case No. 4 demonstrates a multiple group of emotional situations, any one of which, or all collectively, might bear relationship to the stress seen in cases 1 and 3.

Case No. 5 is different from the others in that it is more difficult to demonstrate an exact relationship between the patient's problems on the job and the onset of his illness. However, despite the fact that what was bothering him was not clear, there is no doubt that he had a rather long history of emotional problems in terms of his feelings about work before the onset of multiple sclerosis. This case is particularly interesting because it is the only one that shows a much more chronic process, namely, a period of four years before the onset of the disease.

There are certain characteristics that seem to be shared by the first four patients. They presented evidence of a passive-dependent type of personality, the intensity of which, in terms of dependency needs, became aggravated by the onset of multiple sclerosis. The fifth patient openly resented his passive-dependent position. All of the patients showed rather conspicuous problems of sexual maladjustment and sexual "immaturity." Similarly, the first four patients utilized a "happy-go-lucky" type of superficial personality attribute to mask the sadness and depression evident in their histories and in the observations made by the interviewer. Patient No. 5 was depressed.

Of interest is the fact that these patients had no significant medical or surgical histories prior to the onset of their multiple sclerosis, nor did they display any neurological symptoms or signs prior to the emotional stress that preceeded the onset of their disease. As is fairly typical of many patients who suffer from chronic disease processes, these five patients showed additional stress reenforcement in their histories subsequent to the onset of their condition.

The author urges that more attention be paid to the emotionally traumatic history of the multiple sclerosis patient, as well as to the management of such patients. Many workers who have been interested in the psychiatric aspects of such patients have recorded an impressive amount of experience regarding the psychological problems that attend the management of the patient with multiple sclerosis. It would be beyond the scope of this paper to enumerate them even in terms of bibliography. It is the experience of many people who have worked with multiple sclerosis patients that psychotherapy, in terms of a supportive framework, is of assistance in reducing the exacerbations seen with this disease and has helped to prevent the cyclical pattern frequently associated with this disorder.

REFERENCES

Baldwin, M. V. 1952. "Psychological Aspects of Multiple Sclerosis." *Journal of Nervous and Mental Disorders* 115:299-342.
Borberg, N. C. and V. Zahle. 1946. "Psychopathology of Multiple Sclerosis." *ACTA Psychiatrica et Neurologica* 21:75-89.
Brickner, R. M. and D. J. Simons. 1950. "Emotional Stress in Relation to Attacks of Multiple Sclerosis." *Association for Research in Nervous and Mental Disease: Proceedings (1948)* 38:143-149.
Grinker, R. R., G. C. Haur, and F. P. Robbins. 1950. "Some Psychodynamic Factors in Multiple Sclerosis." *Association for Research in Nervous and Mental Diseases: Proceedings (1948)* 28:456-460.
Harrower, M. R. 1954. "Psychological Factors in Multiple Sclerosis." *New York Academy of Science* 58:715-719.
Harrower, M. R. and V. Kraus. 1951. "Psychologic Studies on Patients with Multiple Sclerosis." *AMA Archives of Neurology and Psychiatry* 66:44-57.
Hollos, S. and Ferenczi. 1925. *Psychoanalysis and the Psychic Disorders of General Paresia*. New York: Nervous and Mental Disease Publishing Company.
Langworthy, O. R. 1948. "Relation of Personality Problems to Onset and Progress of Multiple Sclerosis." *Archives of Neurology and Psychiatry* 59:13-28.
Langworthy, O. R. 1948. "Survey of Maladjustment Problems in Multiple Sclerosis with Possibility of Psychotherapy." *Association for Research in Nervous and Mental Disease: Proceedings (1948)* 28:598-611.
Pratt, R. T. C. 1951. "Investigation of Psychiatric Aspects of Multiple Sclerosis." *Journal of Neurology, Neurosurgery and Psychiatry* 14:326-336.
Voss, G. Jr. 1943. "Psychic Trauma as Pathogenic Factors in Multiple Sclerosis." *Deutsche Med. Schnsclar* 69:255.

Living with Multiple Sclerosis: The Gradual Transition

Florence E. Selder
Kathleen A. Breunig

Multiple sclerosis (MS) is a progressive demyelinating disease of the central nervous system. The disease tends to occur early in life, most commonly between the ages of 20 and 40 and although causation has been speculated upon, few theories have been supported by scientific study. The course of the disease is extremely variable. Diagnostic criteria are poorly defined and frequently the diagnosis is made only after other disease processes have been ruled out.

During the early years of the disease the symptoms often appear and disappear. Further, the course of the disease is variable across individuals. It was thought that it would contribute to our understanding of chronic disease to study persons who have a disease with such great variability. Therefore, a study was designed to answer the question, "What are the reported experiences of persons living with multiple sclerosis?" The method of data collection was intensive interviewing. The sample was obtained from an outpatient neurology clinic located in a large medical center. A list of potential subjects who met the following criteria was considered for the study. The criteria were: (1) diagnosis for a least one year, (2) disease in remission, (3) disease state stable, (4) absence of other chronic disease in exacerbated state, (5) no evidence of mental deterioration or memory loss, and (6) ambulatory or wheelchair status. The study sample was drawn randomly from a list of potential subjects. No age restriction was used. The review boards at the center and at the cooperating university approved the protocol. All subjects agreed to participate in

Florence E. Selder, RN, PhD, is Associate Professor and Urban Research Center Scientist, University of Wisconsin, Milwaukee, WI 53201. Kathleen A. Breunig, RN, MN, is Nursing Supervisor for Ambulatory Care, Zablocki VA Medical Center, Milwaukee, WI 53295.
This research was partly funded by the American Nurses' Foundation.

the study. Data were analyzed using life transition theory as the initial framework. The interviews were transcribed from the audio-tapes. All sentences and paragraphs were assigned codes representing the categories devised from the theory, to allow for retrieval and cross referencing.

SUBJECTS

All 20 subjects were male. The age range was from 38 to 76. All but three subjects completed high school, with eight subjects having more than a high school diploma. Sixteen subjects lived with their spouses and one subject was widowed and lived with his son. The rest of the subjects lived alone. Seven subjects were dependent on others for personal care and the other subjects did their own personal care.

LIFE TRANSITION THEORY

The framework for the study was life transition theory. Data were analyzed using this theory, which evolved from a series of clinical research projects designed to study individuals' responses to disability and chronic illnesses. The theory of life transition concerns the process that bridges from a reality which has been disrupted to a newly constructed or surfacing reality. The emerging reality integrates or incorporates the event(s) or the decision(s) in such a way that the integrity of the person or sense of self is maintained intact. The structuring of the new reality follows expectations held by the person of what that reality should or could become for him or her. The purpose of the structuring is to create new meaning in an individual's life when the old meanings have been fractured.

Life transition theory describes how people restructure their reality and resolve uncertainty, a major characteristic of any transition. The shape of the transition is the resolution of the uncertainty (Selder 1989). For the individuals in this study, reality is disrupted by the occurrence of a chronic disease, multiple sclerosis. The emerging reality is learning to live with the multiple sclerosis. The terminus or closure of the transition is the point when the person attends to aspects in his or her life that no longer center on the disease. It is at that point that other possible life transitions in which the person could engage assume priority over the multiple sclerosis life transition.

GETTING THE DIAGNOSIS

Subjects learned about the diagnosis of multiple sclerosis in a variety of ways. Most frequently, the subjects or their physicians attributed the symptoms of MS to some other disease process. Subjects could, upon reflection, identify their having the symptoms of MS prior to diagnosis. One subject said:

Way back in 1965, I was cutting hair and I never have headaches, never . . . . I got a tremendous headache . . . intense pain . . . I closed my shop . . . I went home . . . it got progressively worse . . . intense high temperature . . . they couldn't discover what was the cause . . . now I think it was the onset of MS . . . however, I went into remission after that. So I didn't think about it again.

Another subject reported:

The first time I noticed it, I was overseas . . . In Africa I got malaria . . . I never paid it any attention, but months before that, I was noticing my legs and my hands. . . . No pain . . . numbness in my legs and arms and I told the doctor that I couldn't pinpoint it . . . now I know.

Those subjects who reported being aware of the symptoms of MS before the disease was diagnosed, attributed these symptoms to overexertion or stress.

One subject said:

Well, I woke up one morning—this was about eight years ago, and I was totally numb from the knees down on both legs, like they were asleep. I had worked pretty hard the day before putting in a sidewalk, and I attributed it to the fact that I had worked hard. So I thought nothing of it. As the day progressed the symptoms didn't go away. As it progressed up my legs to my hips I began to think about, boy, I'd better go to the doctor.

In this study it was common to find that if the symptoms did not persist or progress, then the patient or the physician would ignore them. For instance, one physician said, "Well, I don't know what it is; there's something definitely there, but whenever it comes back, see a neurologist about it." The patient said, "Well, no pain was involved, so I never paid it no mind." Another said, "Well it would come and go, come and go, come and go, and I'd pay no attention to it. Until one day at work my eyes went out; I couldn't see. I said, 'I can't see what I'm doing, I have no business here.' It stayed about a month and then my sight started coming back.''

When the symptoms interfered with a person's activity, and when the symptoms persisted and could no longer be attributed to something in the person's everyday life, then the subject decided to seek medical advice. As one subject said:

> Well, when the numbness didn't subside, it continued and pro-gressed. If it had been just my legs I don't think I would have gone to the doctor. I was very active. I swam a lot. I rode my bike a lot. I golfed a lot. We have three acres of lawn at home and that requires an awful lot of work outside, so I was very active. And I think that in my mind, if it had not progressed past my knees, I wouldn't have gone to a doctor because I would have assumed that normal activity and working would alleviate the problem sooner or later. But, of course, it did progress, and that is the reason I went to the doctor.

A visual disturbance was the symptom that led most reliably to a diag-nosis of multiple sclerosis. A diagnosis was derived much earlier if there was a vision disturbance than if the subjects reported numbness or weak-ness. Further, subjects with visual problems sought medical assistance earlier than subjects with other symptoms. It may be that numbness or weakness can more easily be credited to something other than multiple sclerosis. For instance, one subject said, "Well, I had these symptoms in my back and my legs . . . the back doctor put me in a cast . . . because my legs were dragging . . . it wasn't until a few years later when I went back that he sent me to a neurologist."

Many subjects experienced relief when they were told the diagnosis of MS It may be that during the period of trying to diagnose, the physician would give alternatives that would need to be ruled out before a definitive diagnosis could be made. For instance, one neurologist told a subject, "I haven't evaluated all of the tests yet, but you either have a brain tumor or MS" The subject reported thinking, "Geez, let's hope it isn't a brain tumor because we have a customer who had one removed and he has no sense of taste. At the time I thought that I would choose MS of the two. Had I known then what I know now, I'm very doubtful . . . At least the tumor would have been removable."

LIVING WITH THE DISEASE

Subjects in this study reported that they realized they had the disease and had learned to live with it. When subjects did discuss cures, it was in terms of the benefit for future generations and not for themselves. They viewed the disease as something one fights against. The repeated advice was to do as much as possible for oneself and to keep fighting it. As one subject said, "I don't hold any hope of any great miraculous improvement or anything. I'm just assuming this is what I have, and it's going to progress."

The overall theme in the subjects' description of the transition of living with multiple sclerosis was gradualness. A subject said, "It's a gradual decline, but I'm pretty stable—you always hit those spots in there. The gradual transition, I guess you'd call it, from good health to this health, and you can't live in between, that's how it came about." Another said, "Well, it would come and go, come and go . . . when there's no pain involved, you don't pay any attention. Now, I'm going downhill, slow but sure." And another said, "Well, this thing started with the numbness in the knees . . . rightly eight or nine years ago . . . It has very, well, a good word is inconceivably progressed." Another said, "Very slowly, but it has progressed to the point now where my right leg is almost not operative . . . I swing it when I walk . . . I can't really bend it . . . My left leg is getting there slowly but it still works, so that I can still get around . . . I don't know what else to say . . . only that it's progressing very slowly." Subjects described the transition as progressive and entailing declines.

UNCERTAINTY

The characteristic of the transitions studied has been uncertainty. In this study the major source of uncertainty was fear. All subjects reported fearing that they would be "in bed." The fear was the loss of mobility. Subjects would say that the worst thing that could happen to them would be to be "in bed." Subjects recounted stories of hearing about someone who could only move his head. They did not know how they would handle that. The subjects' uncertainty stemmed from the fear of total dependency.

Subjects uncertainty was confounded by the absence of a specific treatment regimen. Subjects reported using different regimens, and the regimens were not comparable from subject to subject. The variation in the treatment approaches was based on the relationship of the subject to his physician. Typically, a subject reported, "My physician prescribed a fairly well-known relaxant. After I took a pill and a half, I said, this is not for me. I had thought if I relaxed internally a little bit it would help my mobility. It didn't." Another subject said, "I asked my doctor about pills I read about and he said, 'If you'd like to try it that's fine. I tried them and I found no difference so I stopped.' Most subjects have a similar relationship with their doctor, that is, the physician will prescribe what the patient thinks would be helpful and then, if it isn't, the physician stops it.

There was a lot of trying and stopping of treatments. It may be that the use of various treatments reduced uncertainty for the subjects in this study. As one of the subjects reported, "I go to the meetings and these people sit and tell you what they got their physicians to prescribe and I think you have to be careful what you put into your body." Given the unknown nature of the disease, the physician may be placed in a position of giving the patient more control of the medical management of the disease, and if he doesn't, the patient holds the doctor responsible for the results. One subject held his physician responsible for his decline. The subject attributed B_{12} to controlling his MS. He said, "I was doing fine until another neurologist said, 'You're getting too much of that.' I said, 'Wait a minute. With MS, if you get help from anything, stay with it.' He said, 'No, no, no.' Then I went downhill. He wouldn't put me back on it and later when I did get the B_{12} it was too late."

It was thought that remissions would decrease uncertainty. However, subjects reported uncertainty. It may be that remissions were seen as part of the gradualness of the transition. The remissions may be seen as time-outs before the next exacerbation. Remissions did not reduce uncertainty; further, they were viewed as the prelude to the next period that would or could result in additional loss of functions. "In MS," one subject said, "your goals change — not because you want to change, only because you really don't have . . . you're no longer in command of your future per se. I don't know how to explain, you just can't count on it." Another said, "You just normally assume that when you wake up in the morning, everything is going to operate exactly. It doesn't enter your mind, you just assume this, chances are you're right. But I don't know when I go to bed tonight when I wake up tomorrow morning, maybe I can't move my right hand, or my left arm, or maybe I can't get out of bed. I don't know what could happen and so I don't have any goals set . . ."

MANAGING THE DISEASE

Multiple sclerosis is an intrusive disease. It intrudes on one's daily activities and on one's sense of self. For instance, as one subject said, "I can't even cut my meat on my plate. If we go to restaurants, I feel so doggone foolish because my daughter, too, you know, tells the waitress, 'Give me his plate, I'll cut his meat for him.' I feel so doggone foolish because I can't cut the doggone meat. Of course, I can eat by myself yet . . . I just can't use a knife." Another said, "My grandchildren came in and all I could think is get the hell out of here, I didn't say that, but boy, to go to sleep . . . I don't want nothing to do with nobody." Subjects described ways in which they attempted to control the intrusiveness of the disease. Pacing oneself was a way to contain the disease. A key factor in controlling the disease's intrusiveness was in managing fatigue. As one subject reported, "You know that tiredness . . . you can't fight that tiredness. You just got to go to sleep."

Subjects were fearful of the progression of the disease. One said:

> Well, what is important to me is . . . I don't know if you'd call it just reluctance or fear of becoming prostrate. I just don't want to become a thing laying in the bedroom. I may, many many times, push myself too far — there's different schools of thought. Push or don't push. I'm of the school that I'm going to go as long as I can possibly go. I'm going to push myself every day. Sometime during the day I get very tired. Always. Whatever I have to do to keep from becoming something in the bedroom, I'll do it. It doesn't matter what . . . I come home and say, "Hell, I'm tired," and I go to sit down. My second thought almost immediately is — don't sit down.

Subjects in this study took the approach of "being active" as a means to deal with the disease's continuous progression.

Although subjects reported learning to live with the disease, they also reported resenting the disease. One subject said, "The day the man said to me, you have MS . . . utter disgust. I tremendously hate it. It just makes me so angry that I have it. Whatever it does to me, it's going to do to me; I have no control over that." Another said, "Oh, it challenges me . . . but I hate it and I dislike the disease." Another said, "I just don't like it. It embarrasses me. But then I decide that I'm going to do what I'm going to do regardless of the disease but I don't like it. I would like to be like you. I'd like to get up from this chair and just walk, but I can't. And because I can't . . . doesn't mean I'm going to say . . . 'baloney.' I'm not going to do that. I just resent the fact that I can't do it, but it's not going to stop me from doing whatever it is that I want to do . . . maybe it doesn't make sense." Another subject said what he didn't like about the disease was that "It embarrasses me all the time." Subjects described the many instances in which the disease was a source of embarrassment and intrusive to them. Another said, "I accepted the fact a long time ago. I have MS. You make concessions for what you can't do as easily as you could once." All subjects reported a certain resignation. As one person said, "I just can't stress . . . I can't say enough how much I dislike having MS . . . it restricts me. I would give almost anything not to have it. But I do have it, so . . . I have it, I have it. That's all there is to it." The disease intrudes on all aspects of a person's life.

In an effort to contain the disease, subjects make many adjustments in their lives and in their homes. For instance, all subjects had air conditioning in their homes because heat and humidity confounded their symptoms. Subjects made specific adjustments in their daily lives or jobs. For instance, one subject who is a barber said, "The job I have requires a lot of standing . . . so I found a little chair that barbers used many years ago . . . it attaches to the customer's chair and swings around the chair . . . I can take four customers in a row. In terms of pacing, this same subject reported, "On a normal day . . . I sit down after a few customers, or before I get to the next one, then I'm fine and I can go through the whole day."

Adjusting to the disease was important, as it was seen by the subjects as a way to contain the impact of the disease. As one subject reported, "The only thing in my mind is that if MS continues to progress slowly like it has, then maybe if it does, I can adjust as it goes along, and it's not going to be all that bad." Another subject described how he made adjustments: "I bought a golf cart, I have a porto-skoot, I have a wheelchair, I have crutches, every kind of thing to help me continue a normal life, we've got . . . A lot of people don't have these things . . . and can't do certain things because they don't have the aids to help them . . . I'm fortunate."

Adjustments are a way that people can normalize their experiences. Anything that facilitates mobility was welcomed as it normalized the person's daily life. Another way to adjust was to integrate into daily life what could be seen as abnormal occurrences. As one subject reported, "I fall over a lot . . . I have a portable phone . . . if something happens . . . the squad car is sent . . . they pick me up and get me back in my chair . . . they just get me up and leave." This scenario happened several times a month. The person had normalized this occurrence as daily living.

Subjects viewed the adjusting as making concessions. There reportedly was no choice but to adjust. One subject said, "Well, you have to learn to adjust. It's a strange thing, you know, you used to walk over and pick up a bottle and screw the top off and sometimes you just can't do that. You have to make concessions, you have to do it a little differently. You may have to set the bottle on the floor and hold it between your feet . . . you get it done."

The adaptations or adjustments subjects made served to normalize the subjects' experiences. However, this normalization could also be a source of frustration. One subject reported, "I've made adaptations to help me do things that people just do normally. And then you get tired, and it's very difficult, and you get disgusted with yourself. At the same time, you can't project yourself as having problems. If I would tell people I'm just terrible all the time, it wouldn't be long before they would no longer ask me because they don't want to hear all the problems. Besides, everybody's got problems." Therefore, even though the adaptations served to normalize the situation, subjects were then confronted with looking normal but not having the resources to maintain that normal presentation of themselves.

COMPARATIVE TESTING

According to life transition theory (Selder 1989), one process that people engage in as they are dealing with a disruption in their reality is comparative testing. Comparative testing is the process of comparing oneself against an identified role model. In this study, it was posited that other people with multiple sclerosis who have had the disease longer would be the role model for the subjects. However, either because the disease process is not comparable or the models are not adequate, the subjects did not engage in that form of comparative testing. Subjects *did* utilize comparative testing to reduce their uncertainty by looking, not for people who have multiple sclerosis, but for those who have it "worse off." Subjects would say, "Look across the street; you can see somebody worse off than you are . . . there are many guys worse off than I am." It may be that people with multiple sclerosis are too threatened to compare themselves with other persons with MS and so they compare themselves with others whose misfortunes are less threatening.

Several subjects reported, though, that they liked being in a room with people with the same problems, because they were not judged. For instance, if they had to get up and go to the bathroom the others would understand. However, these subjects saw the groups as people telling all their problems. As one person said, "I don't want to go and sit and listen to a man's entire . . . from day one when he first got it through all the medications and this and that . . . I don't want to hear that . . . I really don't want to. I don't want to hear the morbid dialogues on what could or has happened to all of us."

MAKING MEANING

Subjects reported that what they looked forward to were "small pleasures." One man said, "I look forward to my day off and getting up and sitting at the kitchen table and watching the birds and rabbits and drinking coffee all by myself . . . sounds silly. I like doing things but the high point of my week is sitting at the table and straightening out my mind."

Subjects didn't think that the disease made them any stronger or wiser, but they did believe that they were emotionally stronger. They felt that they could withstand some other problems in their lives a little easier than before the disease.

For our subjects, making meaning out of the disease involved learning to live with what they had to the best of their abilities. It meant giving up the thing that they were unable to do. Subjects also looked at living today, because the future was today and not tomorrow. Tomorrow, they said, you could go blind and or your urinary tract "could go" and close doors for you. One said, "You learn not to gloat because if you gloat then you're bananas." The future is limited.

Another way the subjects made meaning was not to give up. As one said:

> I've been fighting it for years. I will never give up . . . I never will. It will be with me until I die. How long that'll be, I don't know. You can't stop it from happening; it happens. There isn't anything that you can do about it. You can't alleviate the problem. You can't stop it from happening. We all have cancer cells within our bodies. They're dormant, but who knows? It could be right at this moment that maybe yours or mine will start to become active. We don't know. So how can you say, "Why did this happen?" It's all a particular set of circumstances that took place which promoted this, whatever it was that triggered it, and this is the end result.

REFERENCE

Selder, F. E. 1989. "Life Transition Theory: The Resolution of Uncertainty." *Nursing and Health Care* 10(8):437-451.

Depression and Adjustment in Friedreich's Ataxia

Michael A. Nigro
Patti L. Peterson

Nicholas Friedreich first described the disorder that today bears his name in 1863. Friedreich's ataxia (FA) is a relentlessly progressive, degenerative neuromuscular disorder that is primarily characterized by ataxia and eventually, cardiomyopathy. The disorder, which is inherited as an autosomal recessive trait, typically presents with appendicular ataxia in middle to late childhood. As the disease progresses, axial ataxia, cerebellar dysarthria, and peripheral neuropathy become apparent. In the later stages of the disease, examination usually reveals normal intellect, dysarthric speech, ocular dysmetria, neurosensory hearing loss, normal motor strength, hypotonia, distal atrophy, pancerebellar signs, prominent posterior column dysfunction, distal diminution to pin sensation, areflexia, and extensor plantar responses. Pes cavus and scoliosis are also commonly seen. Congestive heart failure due to hypertrophic cardiomyopathy is frequently the eventual cause of death and can occur at any age. Glucose and pyruvate intolerance have consistently been observed and resulted in the recent hypotheses that enzymes involved in pyruvate metabolism (i.e., pyruvate dehydrogenase, malic enzyme) are deficient. Currently, the etiology of FA remains unknown.

Several years ago we made the observation that FA patients had an unusually frequent occurrence of severe depression requiring psychiatric intervention. From 1985 to 1987, 32 patients were evaluated for inclusion in a study we conducted regarding the efficacy of amantadine hydrochlo-

Michael A. Nigro, DO, is Director of the MDA Clinic, Michigan Institute for Neurological Disorders, 28595 Orchard Lake Road, Farmington Hills, MI 48018, and is Director of the Department of Neurology, Children's Hospital, Detroit, MI. Patti L. Peterson, MD, is Assistant Professor of Neurology, Children's Hospital, Wayne State University—University Health Center, Detroit, MI 48202.

ride in the symptomatic treatment of the cerebellar dysfunction seen in FA (Peterson, Saad, and Nigro 1988).

In order to pursue the earlier observation regarding an increased incidence of serious depression, the FA patients were also evaluated for the existence of significant depression requiring psychiatric intervention.

Of these 32 patients, four were symptomatic for acute depression and required immediate psychiatric intervention. The patients were either acutely depressed when they came to muscular dystrophy clinic or were hospitalized for medical problems when the depression became apparent. Two patients were suicidal. Long-term antidepressant therapy was required for three patients and all required ongoing psychiatric care. In all patients, the depression manifested with hostility, anorexia, loss of self-worth, guilt, sleep disturbances, and withdrawal. The psychiatric consultant felt all patients suffered an endogenous depression. Superimposed on the endogenous depression were the problems typical of patients with a progressive debilitating disease. Dexamethasone suppression tests were negative. We were unable to identify any factors that distinguished the four depressed patients from the other FA patients. They did not have family histories of depression or bipolar disease, nor were their social situations or physical disabilities significantly different from the other patients. In no patient was a concomitant drug therapy, such as cardiac drugs, deemed responsible for the depression. Computed tomography of the brain, electroencephalography, and evoked potentials did not reveal significant differences between those patients who were depressed and those who were not.

Is endogenous depression more likely to occur in FA patients than in those with other neuromuscular diseases? Is the association of depression and FA real? Four patients out of 32 does not seem a highly significant number; however, in our experience it is disproportionately high. We see over 750 patients a year in our muscular dystrophy clinic. Although our FA population represents 5 percent of this total, it constitutes 40 percent of our patients who suffer severe depression requiring psychiatric intervention. Most patients with neuromuscular disorders other than FA do express difficulty in coping with their disease but do not exhibit signs and symptoms of endogenous depression. Why does the incidence of significant depression appear to be higher in FA? FA differs from the other neuromuscular diseases. FA patients are not weak; despite adequate strength they may be unable to ambulate or perform a simple task such as reaching for a glass of water. The frustration inherent in this type of neurological disability becomes apparent very early on. Does FA involve an inherent organic affective disorder as part of its spectrum of central nervous system involvement? Could it be that depression, in at least some individuals, manifests in this disease because depression is a biochemical disorder, and a putative dysfunctional gene in endogenous depression may be linked to the gene that is abnormal in FA? These questions remain to be answered.

In conclusion, whether or not our observation is correct and if so, what underlies the association, remains to be clarified. Until such time, physicians should be aware of our experience and be ready to provide the necessary psychiatric intervention should one of their FA patients present with signs and symptoms of acute depression. Physicians must also be aware that tricyclic antidepressants have the potential to aggravate preexisting cardiomyopathy and must, therefore, be used with care. We intend to pursue our studies of these patients in an attempt to identify other affected FA patients, to try to determine what distinguishes depressed FA patients from the others, and to better understand the etiology of the depression.

REFERENCE

Peterson, P. L., J. Saad, and M. A. Nigro. 1988. "The Treatment of Friedreich's Ataxia with Amantadine Hydrochloride." *Neurology* 38(9):1478-1480.

Charcot-Marie-Tooth Disease: Disorder or Syndrome?

Robert E. Lovelace

WHAT IS IT?

Charcot-Marie-Tooth disease most commonly affects the extremity muscles of the feet, lower legs and hands so that they slowly become thin and weak. Often the reason that patients consult a doctor is that they develop foot deformities with unstable walking. Most frequently there is a problem with holding the foot up, giving rise to tripping on curbs and the necessity to "step high" and walk deliberately. It is a hereditary disease affecting the peripheral nerves: a neuropathy. As the most common genetic neuropathy it is found in 4 out of 10,000 people. There are at least 125,000 affected patients in the U.S.A.

THE NAME

The name is derived from the three doctors who described the disease over 100 years ago and is commonly abbreviated to CMT disease or disorder. Less commonly it is referred to as "peroneal muscular atrophy" (PMA) describing the thin lower legs which are often referred to as "stork" legs. The name covers a variety of diseases with a similar appearance,[1] but the two common varieties are those with thickened nerves and abnormal fatty (myelin) coverings to the nerve fibers, called Type 1, and those with deterioration of the central axon material of the nerve, called Type 2. Type 1 is sometimes called hypertrophic, and Type 2 neuronal and the commonest hereditary pattern is dominant.

Robert E. Lovelace, MD, is Professor of Neurology, College of Physicians and Surgeons, Columbia University, and Co-Director of the Muscular Dystrophy Clinic, Columbia-Presbyterian Medical Center, New York, NY 10032.

HOW DISABLING?

Life span is not normally reduced by this disease and intellectual ability is equally not affected. Perhaps because of stimulation to achieve, patients often attain considerable social success.[2] Walking difficulties and foot deformities produce the most significant disabilities, and although exceptions exist, most patients are non-athletic and have difficulties with competitive sports and school athletics. Fractures and sprains of ankle and lower legs are therefore not uncommon in uncorrected patients, but only rarely do patients need crutches to walk and only the extremely rare person will be confined to or need a wheelchair. Hands sometimes assume claw like positions and physiotherapeutic aids and procedures may be required in activities of daily living, such as writing, fastening buttons and turning door knobs and screw caps. Although a small percentage of patients with CMT have defects in the cardiac conduction system, such as bundle branch and complete heart block, this is usually not disabling, unlike Friedreich's Ataxia which may resemble CMT and have very serious cardiac disease. Rarely rapid progression may take place during pregnancy, but this usually improves after birth of the baby. If rapid progression occurs otherwise, then additional causes of neuropathy, including immunological diseases, will need to be considered.[3]

AGE OF ONSET

Usually this illness produces foot symptoms during youth or early adult life. However, one variety of the neuronal form (CMT Type 2) can have childhood onset and be extremely disabling.[4] Early features which can be discovered in young children are problems with walking, toe-walking and club feet. In the hypertrophic type the slow conduction velocity characterizing this as Type 1 can be discovered and is established between the ages of 2 and 3 years.[3] At this stage the patient may be relatively asymptomatic. Comments about the neuronal type having a later clinical onset than the hypertrophic type are not born out by all experiences and a distinction cannot be made on this basis.[1]

HOW IS CMT INHERITED?

The common method is by dominant transmission in which it is only necessary for one parent to carry the defective gene, and in these families several generations are often involved. In dominant disorders it is not possible to accurately predict the degree of involvement of affected relatives, which in their children have a 50% chance of having the abnormal gene. This can express itself as a very minor abnormality, pes cavus or a high arched foot without disability or weakness (called "forme-fruste") through moderate involvement with weak and atrophic hands and feet to unsteady and impaired ambulation needing aids. The rarer recessive form needs both parents to have the gene, which in this case usually gives no symptoms in the parents, although if they are blood relatives (consanguineous) this combination is clearly more likely to happen. In comparison with the above (so-called autosomal) inheritance, sex-linked inheritance via the female members only (involving the gene on the X or sex chromosome) in both the recessive and dominant modes has been found to be commoner than previously suspected.[3] Recessive inheritance involves on the average only 25% of the children who are often similar in their clinical manifestations. Clearly, genetic counselling is of great value in this disease. Type 3 (HMSN 3) or Dejerine Sottas disease is rare and is recessive or sporadic, has early onset with prominent sensory manifestations and, like Type 1, has extremely hypertrophic (often visible) and demyelinated nerves with very slow conduction velocity and a pointed face, like a tapir.[3]

DIAGNOSIS

In addition to the clinical evaluation by the physician which will show the characteristic foot, leg and hand weakness with deformities and impaired function in walking and manual manipulation, a thorough investigation of metabolic problems and a point-by-point evaluation of family members is important. Ancillary and often essential studies include neuromuscular electrodiagnosis, commonly called EMG or electromyography. Actually measuring the nerve conduction velocity, even including apparently unaffected blood relatives, is important in establishing the defect and the particular type or variety of CMT. This is non-invasive and likened to a strong tingling sensation with jumping of the muscles. The electromyography is performed by the physician with a very small pointed electrode inserted into various muscles. It confirms and demonstrates the nerve damage or deterioration, as well as separating CMT from other neuromuscular disorders, which may mimic CMT clinically. It is only semi-invasive, the needle being smaller than that used for collecting blood, and when performed by an experienced investigator will only require sedation for young children. Blood and urine studies to evaluate metabolic abnormalities and inborn enzyme defects are important and an electrocardiogram will indicate the infrequent cases with a defect in the heart's conductive system. X-ray, CT scans and MRI (magnetic – non-invasive) will help to evaluate the extremity deformities and spine curvature of scoliosis if present. With our present knowledge, spinal tap with spinal fluid examination and muscle and nerve biopsy may need to be performed in unusual cases with diagnostic problems, but is it generally recommended that these specialized studies be done only in the larger neuromuscular centers with the correct facilities to fully evaluate the material. They are invasive procedures and usually would only need to be performed once.

Interestingly, the unusual cases such as those with spasticity (Type 5), optic atrophy (Type 6), retinitis pigmentosa (Type 7) and other atypical or associated features may make up 30% of our total experience and have the same physical appearance (called the phenotype). They also exhibit a similar range of inheritance patterns, can be entirely distal motor or spinal muscular atrophy with normal motor and sensory conduction (spinal type) or may have a defined storage disorder, such as phytanic acid (a fatty acid) in the recessive disease, Refsum's disease or Type 4.[1,3] The hereditary sensory and autonomic neuropathies usually have much earlier onset but occasionally very similar deformities and are classified as Types 1 to 4,[4] and an extremely severe disease with onset at birth or in early infancy, the congenital hypomyelination syndrome is almost certainly a genetic disorder with similarities to these and the Type 3 or Dejerine Sottas disorder.

TREATMENT AND CURE

Treatment is available, but the possibility of cure awaits the discovery of the abnormal enzyme or biochemical substance produced by the defective gene.

Treatment includes actual treatment of the deformities and walking problems with the help of doctors in rehabilitation medicine and their therapists and also of orthopedic doctors. We have found the help and advice of an experienced podiatrist very valuable with Charcot-Marie-Tooth disease patients. Both appliances and surgery may have a place in management, and the timing of such interventions is a careful judgment call from the primary neuromuscular doctor.

Biochemical abnormalities, particularly those which may cause neuropathy, should be corrected, and in a number of patients who have rapid deterioration appearing to have an immunological basis, appropriate therapy may be useful. This could include "blood washing" or plasmapheresis, and chemical immunosuppression, the latter treatment carrying the risk of side effects. Pregnancy may occasionally be associated with accelerated progress of the disease, and more frequent trips to the primary physicians may be necessary. This is currently under investigation.

The other form of treatment is controlled trials which include gangliosides, hormonal substances and lipid dietary regimens.

RESEARCH

Of course, controlled trials are included under research as are new orthopedic and physiotherapeutic procedures. Other basic research is mainly in the area of molecular genetics where large families, when investigated, can ultimately give valuable information.[3] The Muscular Dystrophy Association and other organizations as well as the neuromuscular centers can provide information of this activity. Several gene locations have been isolated. At a recent symposium held by the Muscular Dystrophy Association, Ionasescu has indicated the possibility of up to six genes being involved on five chromosomes: numbers 1, 9, 15, 17 and X.[4] It is to be hoped that further refinements will make this the diagnostic aide of the future, but until then we need to rely on careful clinical syndrome descriptions leading to research activities. Podiatrists also have research programs in this area. Basic scientists are investigating nerve and myelin development mechanisms as well as evaluating the role of fatty acids and immunological factors.[3]

NOTES

1. Brust, J.C.M., Lovelace R.E., Devi S. Clinical and electrodiagnostic features of Charcot-Marie-Tooth syndrome. *Acta Neurol Scand* 58 (Suppl 68): 1-142, 1978.

2. Lovelace, R.E. "Psychosocial Aspects of Duchenne Muscular Dystrophy Compared with Charcot-Marie-Tooth Syndrome," in *Psychosocial Aspects of Muscular Dystrophy and Allied Diseases: Commitment to Life, Health and Function*, edit L. Charash, S. Wolf, A.H. Kutscher, R.E. Lovelace and M. Hale: 1-12, 1983.

3. *Charcot-Marie-Tooth Disorders: Pathophysiology, Molecular Genetics, and Therapy*: edit R.E. Lovelace and H.S. Shapiro, Publ. Wiley-Liss, New York, January, 1990.

4. Lovelace, R.E. Hereditary Induced Peripheral Neuropathies, in *Clinics in Podiatric Medicine and Surgery*, edit. G. Weber, Vol. 7 #1, pp. 37-50, 1990.

Psychosocial Aspects
of Charcot-Marie-Tooth Disease
in Childhood

Linda Phillips Goldfarb
Howard K. Shapiro

For most people, childhood and adolescence are carefree times. For a child with a disability, this may not always be the case. A child with a disability such as Charcot-Marie-Tooth syndrome (CMT) may have a whole set of worries and concerns that would never enter the mind of an ordinary, healthy child. As the clinical symptoms of this genetic peripheral neuropathy develop, muscle wasting is most apparent in the lower leg and forearms. Physical coordination decreases and a child's lifestyle is affected in many ways.

This study was based on interviews with twenty adult CMT patients (ten male and ten female) with regard to their childhood and adolescent experiences. For most of these people the age of clinical onset was in the first or second decade. That is to say, their disability began to become apparent before the age of 20 (Figure 1). Most reported that the degree of severity during childhood/adolescence ranged from what they described as mild to bad (Figure 1). All study participants were confirmed to have Charcot-Marie-Tooth syndrome, also known as peroneal muscular atrophy, by previous clinical examination. However, patients were not further classified as to electrophysiological or genetic subvarieties of this syndrome.

Linda Phillips Goldfarb is Coordinator, New York Chapter, National Foundation for Peroneal Muscular Atrophy, 240 East 27th Street, New York, NY 10016. Howard Shapiro, PhD, is Director of Scientific Program, National Foundation for Peroneal Muscular Atrophy, University Science Center, 3624 Market Street, Philadelphia, PA 19104.

The authors wish to thank Lauren Ugell for her assistance in survey work on this study.

109

FIGURE 1. (A) Age of CMT clinical symptom onset as described by 20 patients, (B) degree of clinical severity during childhood/adolescent years as assessed by patients.

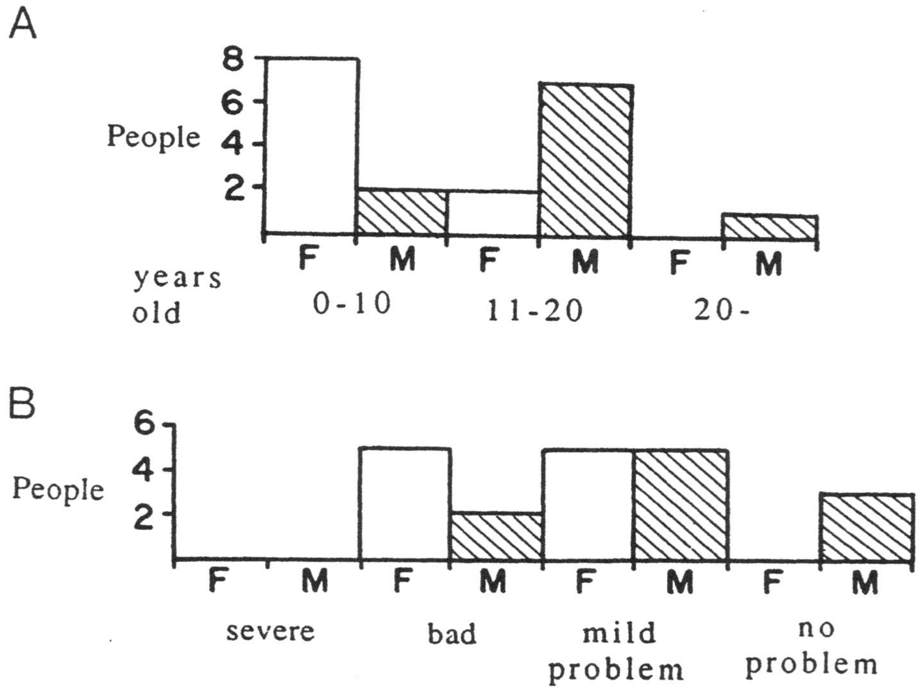

As noted in Figure 1 and other data (see below) there appeared to be a tendency for male interviewees to play down the role of CMT in their childhood. To explore this question our interview protocol included a request for patients to describe the degree of pain and discomfort they experienced during electromyographic testing (Figure 2). This form of neurological testing involves application of electrical stimulation to nerves of the arms and legs. There is nothing about the physical nerve responses to this test that would be different for males or females. Yet, as shown in Figure 2, our male subjects tended to describe electromyographic tests as being somewhat less painful. The general inclination of males in our study to understate their emotional feelings appeared in their responses to many of our questions. This gender-specific response phenomenon has been observed in other psychosocial studies (Steward and Lykes 1985).

Most of the women and some of the men felt that having CMT had affected their self-image (Figure 3). Several people said that they were never able to meet their parents' expectations. One of the women said, "My mother expected me to do everything; learn to ride a bike, rollerskate, play tennis and so on. I failed miserably at all of them. My mother has the disease as well, but she must have felt great guilt for passing it on to me. As a result, I always felt that it was my fault, that I just didn't try hard enough."

Pursuing the question of self-image, we also asked our study participants about their sense of body image during childhood and adolescence (Figure 4A). During childhood our female interviewees were evenly divided regarding CMT as a major factor, minor factor, or no factor in body image. During adolescence females actually tended to feel that CMT was a smaller factor in appraising body image. In accord with generally accepted definitions of sex roles, women were less concerned about developing physical strength and sports abilities during adolescence. Male responses concerning body image also seemed to fit in with generally accepted definitions of sex roles. During childhood almost all males interviewed felt that CMT had become a major factor in their sense of body image.

We also asked our study participants how CMT affected their sense of masculinity/femininity during adolescence. The response pattern was exactly that seen when we questioned them regarding their adolescent sense of body image (Figure 4B). Although CMT tended to become an issue in adolescent self-appraisal, as seen in Figure 5, it seemed to have little direct effect on dating. For most of our interviewees, CMT was not a significant problem regarding teenage dating.

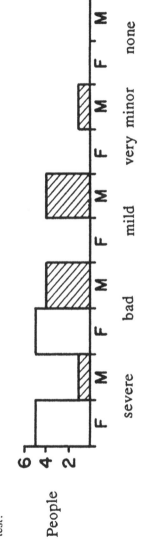

FIGURE 2. Twenty CMT patients who had undergone neurological testing were asked, "Have you ever had an electromyography test? If so, how would you rate the degree of pain and discomfort during the test?"

FIGURE 3. Patients were asked (A) "During childhood did CMT affect your self-image?" and (B) "During adolescence did CMT affect your self-image?"

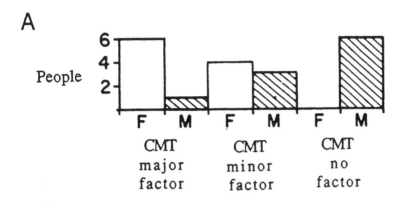

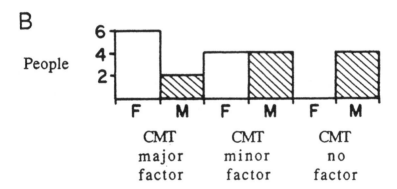

Half of the subjects said that having the disease caused them to feel apprehensive about school (Figure 6). Several people noted that they were afraid to raise their hand in class, as they did not wish to focus attention on themselves and their disability. A few also said that they had become introverted. Part of the problem may lie in the fact that teachers frequently misunderstand this disability.

More than half of our interviewees admitted that their relationships with peers were somewhat affected. Fifteen out of 20 said that they felt "different" (Figure 7A). Yet only one quarter of these people said CMT was a major factor in how they were actually treated by peers during high school (Figure 7B). One woman said, "I felt that the friends who chose me were

FIGURE 4. Patients were asked (A) "During childhood did CMT affect your sense of body image?" and (B) "During adolescence did CMT affect your sense of body image?"

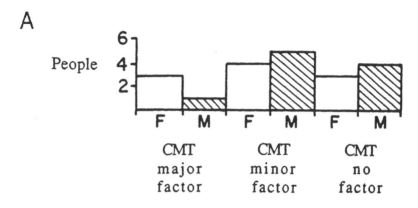

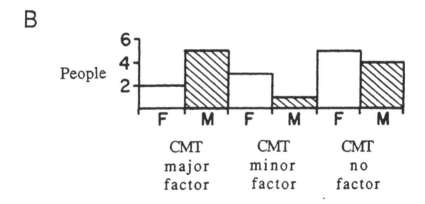

not really the 'top people' or they would not have chosen me. If they knew what I was really like, they would have dropped me. In college I was quite popular, and I questioned what was wrong with these people. Couldn't they see that I was a 'subperson'?" Another woman said, "I was ashamed of being unable to go up steps without railings. So I did not participate in certain activities. I could not explain or talk about it and I became more introverted."

When asked how CMT in general affected their high school experiences, half of our female and one-third of our male subjects said that CMT was a major factor (Figure 8). Many said that gym was a particular problem. Four of our subjects were forced to stop taking gym class because of their CMT (Figure 9A). Many reported that participation in gymnastic activities was a notable source of anxiety.

One man said, "Gym was very embarrassing. The teachers didn't believe that I had a physical problem and I was expected to do what everyone else could do. One gym teacher tried to degrade me in front of the rest of the class."

Among those who could participate in sports, none did particularly well. "I was always the last to be chosen for any team" was a frequent response. Several people said that they were good swimmers. Many described themselves as clumsy. One man said, "My father and brothers were all good baseball players. I could never measure up to them. I felt that it was my fault, that I was just being lazy!"

FIGURE 5. Patients were asked "During your adolescent years was CMT a problem regarding dating?"

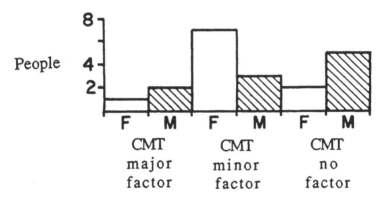

FIGURE 6. Patients were asked "Did CMT create apprehension toward elementary/high school?"

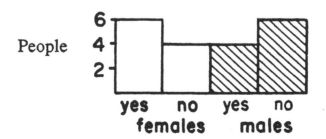

FIGURE 7. Patients were asked (A) "Did you feel 'different' during elementary/ high school?" and (B) "How were you treated among friends and peers during high school?"

A

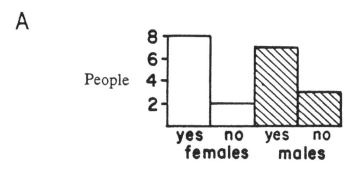

B

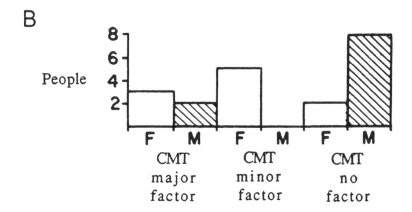

When asked if they had "overcompensated" in other areas because of their physical limitations, many reported that they had (Figure 10). Many had done well academically and several listed other nonphysical activities. One man reported that he had meticulously built model ships, which was a challenge in light of his hand tremor.

Our survey found no indications of impaired intellectual function. Three-quarters of our study participants had at least some college education (Figure 11A). Of these 15 people, only three described CMT as a major factor during their college years (Figure 11B). Yet when asked if they would have chosen a different career if they did not have CMT, one-

FIGURE 8. Patients were asked, "Regarding CMT, what was high school like?"

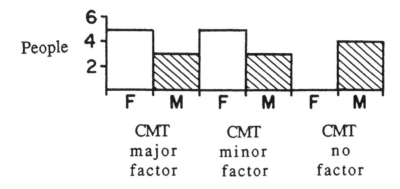

third of the females and almost half of the males said that they would have.

When questioned about their general state of mind during their growing up years, more than half of our subjects described CMT as a major cause of anxiety, frustration and insecurity (Figure 12). For half of the females CMT was also a major source of anger, humiliation and feelings of denial regarding their disability (Figure 13). Fear, depression and guilt were strong feelings in about one third of the females (Figure 14).

One person noted, "Always having to look for ways of getting around physical barriers put one in a constant state of anxiety." While another person recalled, "Going anywhere was such a chore that the tension and anxiety took away the joy of what I was going to do. I was drained from anticipation, fear and anxiety from planning which way to go." One woman was never able to speak with her father, from whom she had inherited CMT, about her fears regarding the progression of the disease. Her father simply could not deal with it. Two women who were interviewed mentioned that they had entertained thoughts of suicide in adolescence. The tendency of males to understate their feelings was readily apparent in the survey questions summarized in Figures 12, 13 and 14.

When considering the findings of this study, one should keep in mind that CMT syndrome presents with a considerable amount of clinical heterogeneity. This means, quite simply, that some patients are far more affected than others. Some patients are not aware of a neuromuscular problem until late adolescence or adulthood. Others, even in the same family, may be crippled outright early in childhood. The wide spectrum of psychosocial problems described in our work in part reflects that we are

FIGURE 9. Patients were asked (A) "Did you take gym class in elementary/high school?" and (B) " Did participation in gym class create anxiety during elementary/high school?

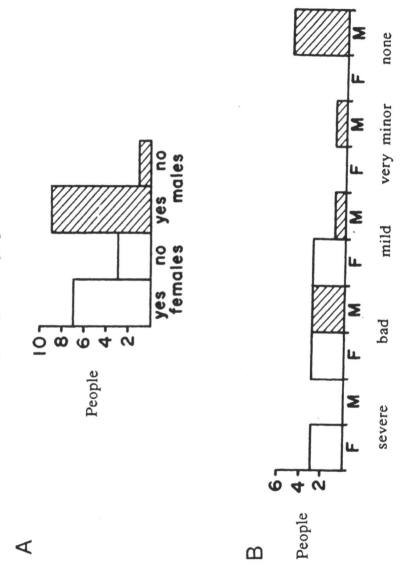

describing people having a wide range of functional loss. In addition, people respond differently to the onset of a physical disability. Some see it as a challenge, something that can be confronted and overcome in many ways. Others, faced with the same functional loss or less, may feel personally defeated.

It should be noted that this was only a preliminary study and, should a more definitive follow-up study be done, it would be desirable to strictly classify people in terms of their clinical status. We did not have access to the medical records of our subjects. It should also be noted that many of the women in our study reported age of onset as being in the first decade. This is contrary to many statements in the medical literature, which describe typical onset, regardless of gender, as being in the second decade or later.

We have concluded from our study that the childhood of a person with a neuromuscular disease such as CMT is clearly fraught with a host of psychosocial problems not experienced by the healthy child. For children with this disease, the psychosocial implications of their disability may broadly affect their lives, involving their school activities, relationships with peers, and participation in sports. For the adolescent patient, the effects of their disability may be extended to become a factor in their social life, i.e., dating. In addition, for the adolescent patient, CMT may become a factor in career planning. We saw nothing in our data to indicate that CMT was a direct limitation on academic performance. In fact, many patients will overcompensate for their disability by actively pursuing other activities not limited by their physical problems.

A key issue facing parents of CMT children and medical professionals is when and how to explain to a child that he or she is developing a

FIGURE 10. Patients were asked "During adolescence do you think that you overcompensated in other areas because of your physical limitations?"

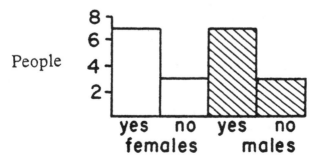

FIGURE 11. Patients were asked (A) "Did you have any college education?" and (B) "If so, what were your college years like regarding CMT?"

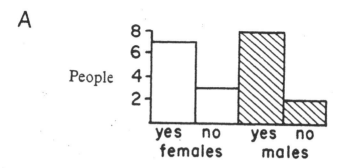

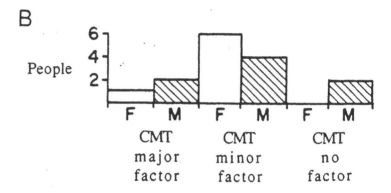

functional disability. Many times, especially in families where other CMT cases have already been diagnosed, parents become aware that a child is developing initial clinical symptoms. Such initial symptoms may include clumsiness, a "lazy" walking gait, difficulty running, tiring easily, changes in the way a child holds a pen or pencil, frequent tripping and ankle sprains, and changes in foot bone structure, such as development of high arches or hammertoes.

In our experience, there is no reason why children cannot be told of their disability. What is most important is the attitude of the parents and medical professionals. Children are very aware of signs of stress and anxiety in their parents' behavior. Likewise, medical professionals may also overreact, behaving as if there is much terrible information that must be kept hidden. This sends children the wrong message. How a child is in-

FIGURE 12. Patients were asked to evaluate their CMT disability as a source of (A) anxiety, (B) frustration or (C) insecurity during their growing up years.

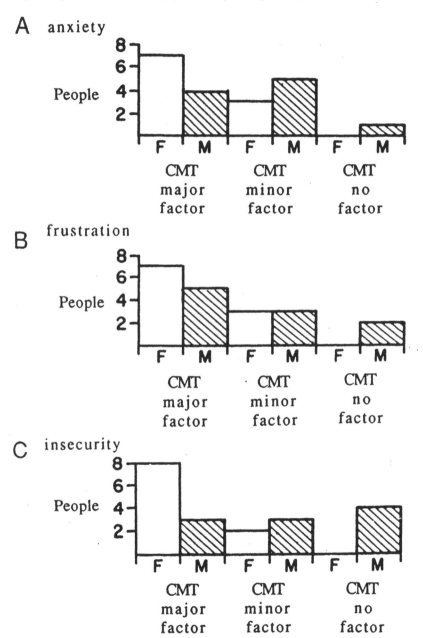

FIGURE 13. Patients were asked to evaluate their CMT disability as a source of (A) anger, (B) humiliation or (C) denial during their growing up years.

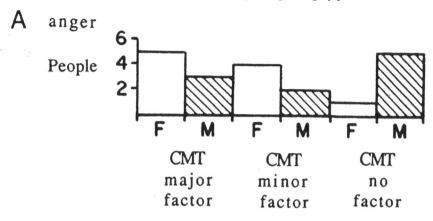

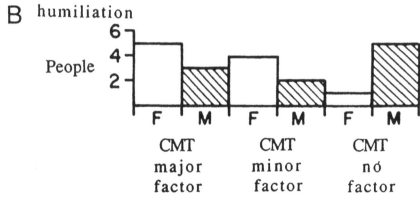

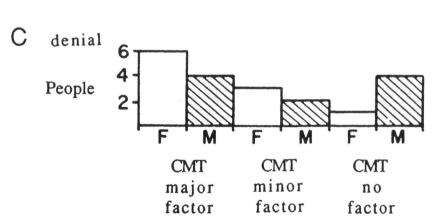

FIGURE 14. Patients were asked to evaluate their CMT disability as a source of (A) fear, (B) depression or (C) guilt during their growing up years.

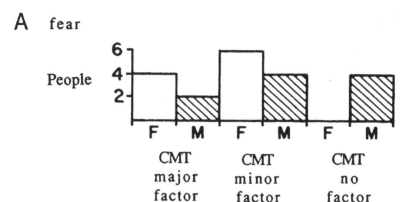

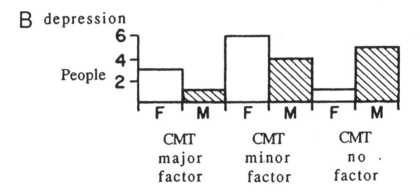

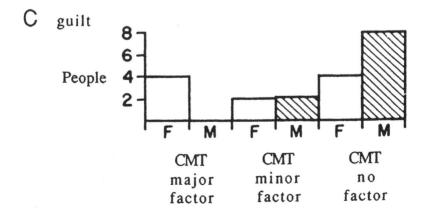

formed that he or she has a recognized medical disability and how he/she is treated subsequently by parents has a great effect on the child's self image and expectations.

When discussing such an issue with children it is important to keep one's approach low key. Yes, the youngster does have a problem. He or she may not excel in sports, but life can and will go on. His or her intellectual ability will not be affected. These children may do quite well in school and have many career opportunities. Their life expectancy is normal. They will have some limitations, but in most ways they can simply go on with their lives. If one of the parents is a CMT patient, hopefully he or she is setting this kind of example.

REFERENCE

Stewart, A. J. and M. B. Lykes. 1985. *Gender and Personality*. Durham, NC: Duke University Press.

Psychosocial Aspects
of Charcot-Marie-Tooth Disease
in the Adult Patient

Howard K. Shapiro
Linda Phillips Goldfarb

As Charcot-Marie-Tooth syndrome (CMT) is a chronic, progressive neuromuscular disease, the clinical symptoms become more apparent as patients reach adulthood. Patients who had minor disabilities during their growing years now are more likely to encounter problems with walking, writing, balance, chronic pain, and stamina. Patients who had relatively advanced CMT symptoms during childhood may face quite serious limitations on their lives. In addition to damage to peripheral motor and sensory nerves, CMT patients also experience some loss of autonomic nervous system function. These nerve fibers regulate normal automatic body functions such as breathing, heart rate, sweating, peristaltic movement of food through the digestive tract, the action of stomach sphincters (valves), and sexual response. Some nerve damage, generally limited, may become apparent in any combination of these nerve functions in CMT patients. To explore the psychosocial aspects of CMT on adults we surveyed 20 patients (10 males and 10 females). These individuals were not previously interviewed for either our study of CMT during childhood or our study of the CMT family.

As in our childhood/adolescence study, 20 patients in this survey who had undergone diagnostic testing by electromyography (EMG) were asked to evaluate the degree of discomfort they experienced. As seen in our childhood/adolescence study, male patients were more likely to describe

Howard Shapiro, PhD, is Director of Scientific Program, National Foundation for Peroneal Muscular Atrophy, University Science Center, 3624 Market Street, Philadelphia, PA 19104. Linda Phillips Goldfarb is Coordinator, New York Chapter, National Foundation for Peroneal Muscular Atrophy, 240 East 27th Street, New York, NY 10016.

the pain and discomfort of EMG testing as mild or very minor, while female patients were much more likely to describe the pain as severe or bad (Figure 1). The EMG test involves use of diagnostic equipment that applies pulses of electrical current to the arms and legs. There is, in fact, some physical pain and discomfort involved in taking this test, but the laboratory procedure and the physical response of those being tested are the same regardless of gender. Hence the findings shown in Figure 1, like the corresponding findings in our childhood/adolescence study, suggest that male interviewees tended to understate their personal evaluations of this aspect of their disability.

Typical of this gender difference in responses is the data shown in Figure 2. When CMT patients were asked when their physical symptoms first became apparent, females tended to describe clinical onset during childhood, while males were far more likely to describe clinical onset during adolescence or adulthood. This gender-specific discrepancy in response is in contradiction to neurological findings reported in the medical literature (Bird and Kraft, 1978). It appears that men did not consider their disease to be a problem until more overt symptoms began to appear, such as difficulty climbing stairs.

Some introductory lifestyle questions gave us an overview of the role of CMT in these peoples' lives. As shown in Figure 3, more than half of our female subjects described CMT as a major factor in day-to-day living. One-third of the women noted that CMT seriously limited their ability to do household chores, while the majority of men felt that CMT had little or no limiting effect. Half of the female interviewees felt that their CMT seriously limited their ability to do shopping chores (Figure 4A). In a related question (Figure 4B), half of the women who had learned how to drive noted that CMT either limited their driving ability or prevented them outright from driving. Some of those patients still able to drive required special hand controls for their cars.

Regarding her day-to-day activities, one woman said, "I have to plan everything I do in advance. I have to get up much earlier than other people in order to get a parking spot close to my office." Another woman who has difficulty with hand function reported that before she goes shopping she approximates what she is going to spend in every store and sets up her bills with paper clips to avoid having to fumble around in her wallet. Many said that they had to plan out every day in advance, carefully pacing themselves to avoid fatigue. A woman who lives in a major city said, "I wear leg braces that are rigid. I cannot take buses and subways because of the steps. I am dependent on cabs to go any distance and I can't find one

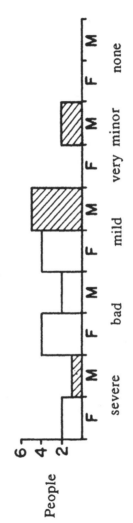

FIGURE 1. Twenty patients having Charcot-Marie-Tooth syndrome who had undergone diagnostic testing by electromyography were asked, "How would you rate the degree of pain and discomfort that you experienced during your electromyography test?

FIGURE 2. Patients were asked "What was your age of CMT clinical onset?"

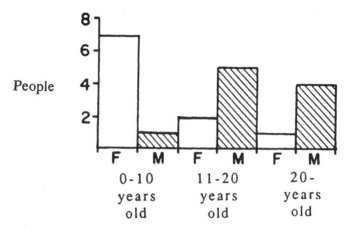

before 10:00 AM. I know that I can not make appointments before 10:30 AM. I have to plan my appointments so that I am not in very crowded areas at peak hours. I don't get around that well and I fear being knocked over in a crowd." Another woman said that she has learned to do much of her shopping through catalogues.

We found that self-image was affected to some extent, as was the way that people viewed their bodies with regard to the disease (Figure 5). Half of the people said that having the disease had no bearing on their feelings of masculinity or femininity. However, a few people made comments such as, "I would feel more feminine if I could put on an attractive pair of shoes. People say, 'You dress so well, but look at your shoes!' " or "I wear braces. I think that my boyfriend would really like to see me in high heels and a miniskirt!" "I don't see myself as feminine, because being feminine, to me, means being graceful, and I am clumsy."

Turning our attention to peer relationships, we asked the patients in our study group several questions regarding CMT as an issue for their friends. Very few adults had difficulty in discussing the disease with their friends; similarly, very few of their friends had difficulty in discussing the disease with them (Figure 6). However, many people felt that CMT did in fact limit their activities with friends (Figure 7). Only five people were still able to dance without difficulty. One man reported that he loved to dance. He and his wife had taken dancing lessons, but he had to give it up. He now can only dance slow dances, while holding on to his wife for balance. A young woman who likes to go to discos reported that she was glad that

FIGURE 3. Patients were asked (A) "To what extent has CMT affected your day-to-day living?" and (B) "Has CMT limited your ability to do household chores?"

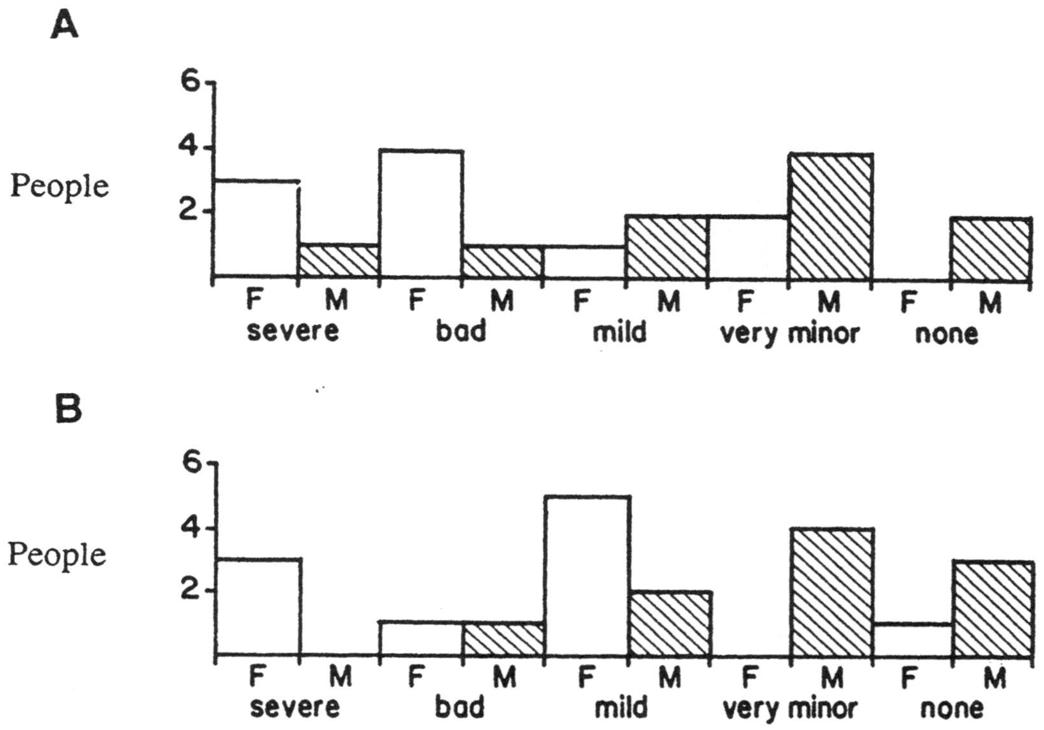

FIGURE 4. Patients were asked (A) "Has CMT limited your ability to do shopping chores?" and (B) "To what extent, if any, has CMT affected your ability to drive a car?"

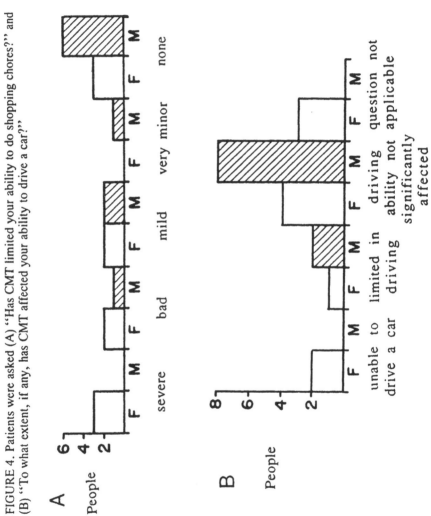

FIGURE 5. Patients were asked (A) "How has CMT affected your self image during your adult years?" (B) "As an adult, does having CMT affect the way you feel about your body?" and (C) "In your adult years, does having CMT affect your feelings of masculinity or femininity?"

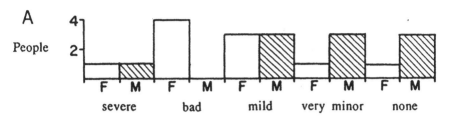

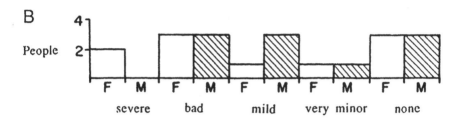

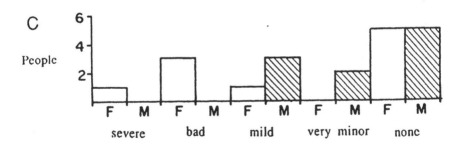

free style dancing was back in style. She said that she used to fear that her partner would swing her out and she would lose her balance.

Several of our questions dealt with education and career choices. Higher education does not appear to have been limited by the presence of CMT, as seen in Figure 8. This suggests that intelligence was not affected in these individuals. Yet, for some of our interviewees, the presence of

FIGURE 6. Patients were asked (A) "Do you have difficulty discussing CMT with your friends?" and (B) "Do your friends have difficulty discussing CMT with you?"

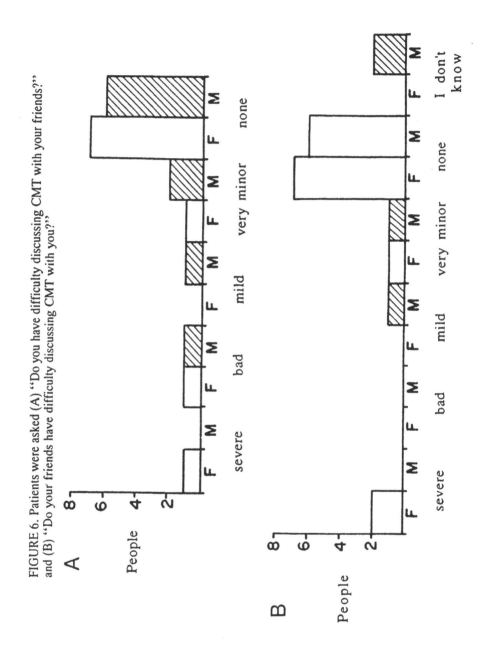

FIGURE 7. Patients were asked (A) "To what extent does you physical disability limit your activities with friends", and (B) "Are you able to dance now?"

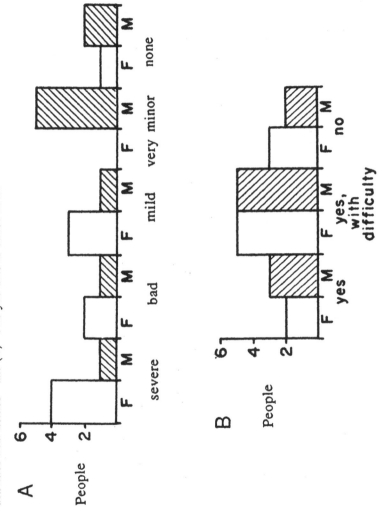

FIGURE 8. Educational background of the CMT patients in our adult psychosocial study.

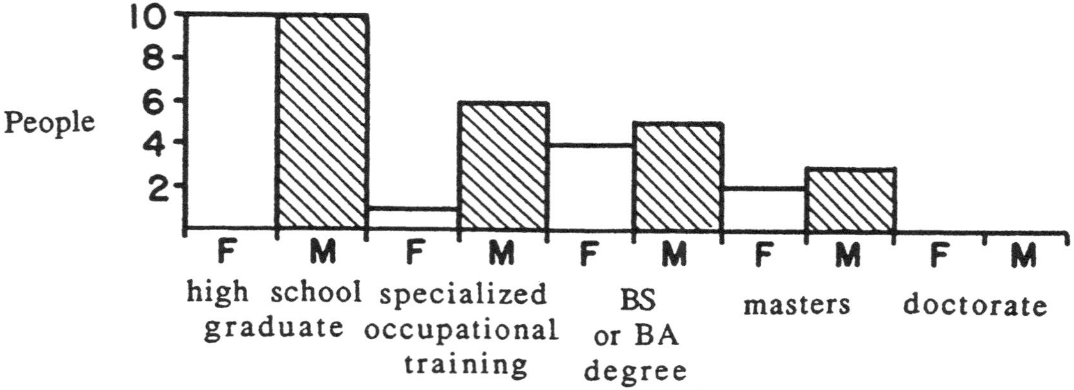

CMT was an important factor in choosing a career and forced approximately one-third of our subjects to change their careers (Figure 9). For example, a man who is a maintenance supervisor is now limited to doing special nonphysical tasks such as training others. A woman who was a biology teacher now works as a laboratory specialist. (Standing all day and having to constantly raise her hand above her head to write on the blackboard had become too difficult.) She also found that having to grade papers after school was too much work, as she suffers from extreme fatigue.

Most of the people who were interviewed said that their disability was generally known among their colleagues at work. When questioned about disability discrimination at work, most people reported that this was not a

FIGURE 9. Patients were asked (A) "Has the presence of CMT been a determining factor in your choice of career?" and (B) "Have you had to change your career because of CMT?"

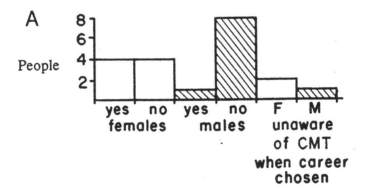

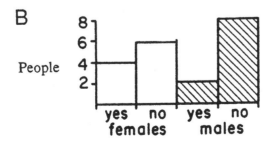

problem. However, one woman had a different story. She worked in a city government building. To enter it, she had to climb a steep set of steps with no hand rails. She was able to enter the building by having a co-worker meet her every morning and help her up the stairs. This woman wrote numerous letters to government officials and was eventually able to get the attention of a local congressman, who ultimately had railings installed.

When asked what role various feelings play in their adult lives, patients most frequently described CMT as a source of frustration, fear, and anxiety (Figure 10). Frustration seemed to be a common problem. One said, "People assume that we can do what anyone else can do because we look so normal, and often we can't." A man who is an electrician gets very frustrated at times when tools drop out of his hands.

For about one-quarter of our interviewees, CMT was also a major source of anger, depression, and insecurity (Figure 11). However, feelings of denial (toward the existence of their disability), guilt, and humiliation about their disability were generally not major factors in the adult lives of our study subjects (Figure 12). It is important to note that not all of our subjects' feelings about their disability were negative. One woman said, "I think that having this disease has given me courage, strength, and determination." This attitude of emotionally overcoming one's disability appears to be widespread among CMT patients.

The issue of family planning was discussed in several ways. Very few people had chosen not to have children, although CMT is a class of inherited disorders (Figure 13). Some study subjects acknowledged that they had chosen to limit the size of their families because of CMT. Patients clearly had difficulty discussing this subject. On the question of limiting family size, eight of 10 women either chose not to answer or, because they had not married, stated that the question was not applicable.

Theoretical questions regarding possible use of a CMT prenatal screening test appeared to be the most personally difficult questions of our study. At this time no prenatal screening test for CMT disorders is available. Such clinical tests may not be available for many years, as research on this subject is still in its initial stages. Yet the issue of possible use of such a test is a most stressful question for CMT patients. If such a test was available, the patients in our study were divided about whether they would want to use it (Figure 14). Here again, many women stated either that the question was not applicable or that they simply chose not to respond. The most difficult of these theoretical questions was whether a positive result on a CMT prenatal screening test would influence a person's decision to proceed with an abortion. Our interviewees were most divided on this

FIGURE 10. Patients were asked to evaluate their CMT disability as a source of (A) frustration, (B) fear or (C) anxiety during their adult years.

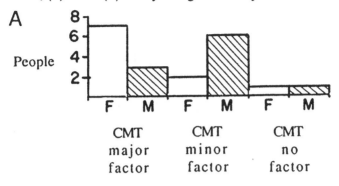

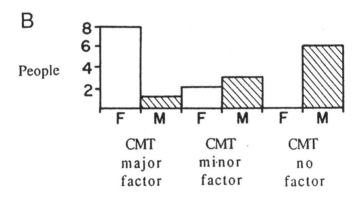

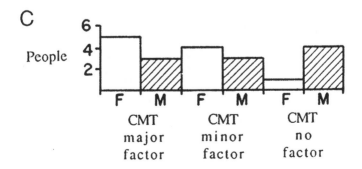

FIGURE 11. Patients were asked to evaluate their CMT disability as a source of (A) anger, (B) depression or (C) insecurity during their adult years.

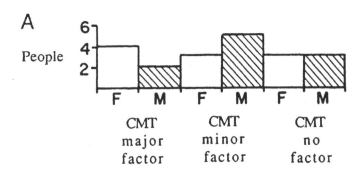

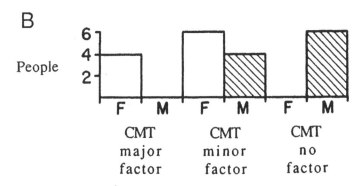

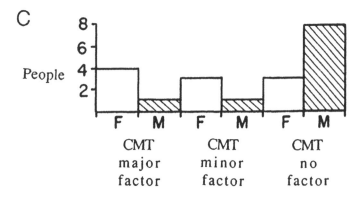

FIGURE 12. Patients were asked to evaluate their CMT disability as a source of (A) denial, (B) guilt or (C) humiliation during their adult years.

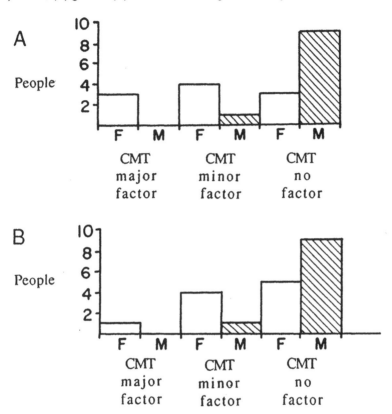

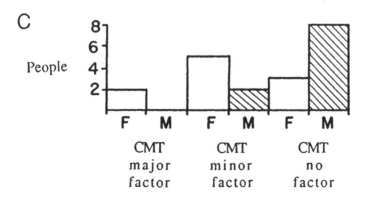

FIGURE 13. Patients were asked (A) "Because of CMT, have you chosen not to have children?" and (B) "Because of CMT, have you chosen to limit the number of children you have or plan to have?"

A

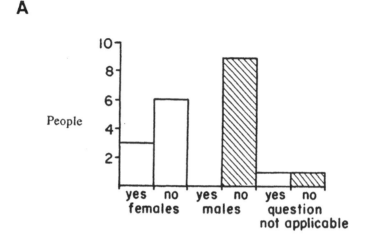

B

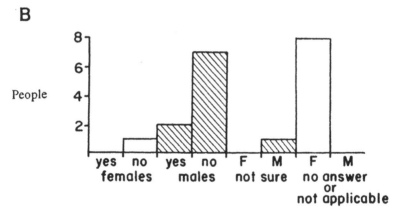

question (Figure 14) as it encompassed two difficult issues, the question of abortion and the question of knowingly passing a genetic disease to one's offspring.

For most of the adult patients interviewed for this study, CMT has had broad and multifaceted effects on their lifestyles, bearing on family relationships, career decisions and a variety of other aspects affecting their personal lives. Many patients have had to face these problems virtually

FIGURE 14. Patients were asked (A) "If a CMT prenatal screening test was available, would you want to use it?" and (B) "If a prenatal CMT screening test was available, would results indicating that the fetus had CMT affect your decision to abort or not abort the pregnancy?"

(A)

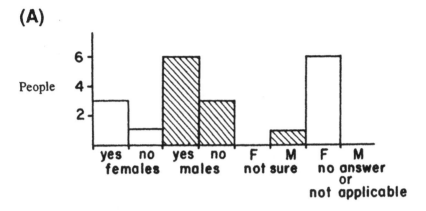

(B)

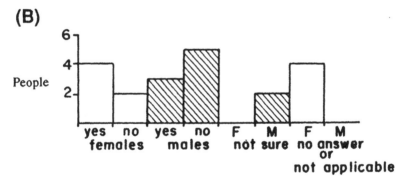

alone. Along the way they have encountered medical professionals who knew nothing about their disease, medical professionals who gave them incorrect advice, and family members, friends, and colleagues who could not understand their disability.

Accurate, practical information on CMT has been sadly lacking within the medical community. This is the most common genetic neurological syndrome, affecting approximately 125,000 Americans. It should be recognized as the public health issue it really is.

CMT patients can make many adjustments in their personal lives to make living with their disability easier. Yet, in closing, we may note two practical issues that tend to have long-term negative effects on their lives: medical insurance discrimination and forced career changes. Over an extended period of time, both of these factors tend to force CMT patients into poverty. Many CMT patients may go on for years without requiring special medical attention, but neurological testing, leg braces, orthopedic surgery and physical therapy can be significant medical costs. When it comes to the attention of an insurance company that someone has CMT, there is a distinct possibility that he or she will not be offered a comprehensive medical policy. Many CMT patients are unable to obtain adequate medical insurance. As of now this issue remains unresolved.

As their disability becomes more advanced, many CMT patients must make career changes. This may involve periods of unemployment and, ultimately, a new job with a lower salary. For some people, being forced out of their career during midlife means forced early retirement and government medical disability support.

With proper medical care, understanding from their families, and prudent career planning, CMT patients can live full, well-adjusted adult lives. Awareness of this public health issue within the medical community is starting to grow and practical medical advice is becoming more available. CMT patients face many challenges, but in many ways these challenges can be met.

REFERENCE

Bird, T. D. and G. H. Kraft. 1978. "Charcot-Marie-Tooth Disease: Data for Genetic Counseling Relating Age to Risk." *Clinical Genetics* 14(1):43-49.

Charcot-Marie-Tooth Disease and the Family: Psychosocial Aspects

Ann Lee Beyer
Teresa Daino

Unlike some dystrophies such as Duchenne, amyotropic lateral sclerosis or some forms of Friederich's ataxia, Charcot-Marie-Tooth disease (CMT) or peroneal muscular atrophy is not fatal and therefore is often dismissed by the medical community as a benign disease. Compared with other neuromuscular diseases, it does indeed appear to be benign, but those who have it consider it to be neither dismissible nor benign.

People who have CMT do suffer. E. J. Cassell states that "suffering occurs when an impending destruction of the person is perceived; it continues until the threat of disintegration has passed or until the integrity of the person can be restored in some other manner" (1982, p. 640). Suffering is not just physical but has to do with the whole person and includes how one perceives oneself, relationships with others, and how one fits into and is able to function in society. Even though a progressive neuromuscular disease is not fatal, it can impose physical and emotional limitations, and the threat of disintegration always exists.

Those with CMT have additional suffering. Very little is known about this hereditary disease and it often takes years to get a correct diagnosis. According to The Foundation For Peroneal Muscular Atrophy (1987, p. 1), people are ". . . too often misdiagnosed, frequently misunderstood, and repeatedly misdirected." There is no cure, and, like most other nonfatal rare diseases, it generates little research. In its milder stages CMT often requires the need for surgery and braces. In its more severe stages it can cripple.

Ann Lee Beyer is Coordinator, New Jersey Chapter, National Foundation for Peroneal Muscular Atrophy, 18 Brownstone Way, Upper Saddle River, NJ 07458. Teresa Daino is a volunteer at the same institution.

143

Even when they are properly and timely diagnosed, people often feel isolated as most of them do not know anyone else with this disease, or for that matter, anyone who has even heard of it. Even its name creates problems in that it implies a dental rather than a neuromuscular affliction. People tell us that because of this, it is often difficult to explain what it is they have.

Almost nothing is known about how CMT affects individuals' lives or how it affects families. Even less is known about how people deal with it. Anthropologist Robert Murphy, who has just written an outstanding book on what it is like to be disabled in our society, has lamented that one of the questions a person with a disability or illness is never asked by physicians is, what is it like (1987, pp. 87-88). This is a question that anthropologists, whose concern is the whole person, often ask. It might contribute to the understanding of CMT if physicians also asked patients that question. As Cassell points out, "Personhood has many facets and it is ignorance of them that actively contributes to the person's suffering" (1982, p. 640). This preliminary study is an attempt to look at a rare disease and ask the question, what it is like to have Charcot-Marie-Tooth disease?

We were interested in both parents and children as individuals, as members of families, and also as members of society. When a member of a family or community has a chronic illness, it affects everyone, and everyone, in turn, has an impact on how the individual handles his or her disease. This includes both other family members and society as a whole, including the medical community. When that disease is rare, hereditary, and can result in a progressive loss of function, the issues become rather complex.

Interviews were conducted with 22 parents in families in which a child has been diagnosed with the disease. The respondents were taken from two support groups for people who either have CMT or have a family member with it. In 15 of these families a parent also had CMT.

Our survey was modeled on Leventhal's "Psychosocial Assessment of Children With Chronic Physical Disease" (1984) and applied to families with CMT. We were interested in:

1. Which family member has the disease;
2. The severity of the disease and its complications;
3. The effects of the disease on:

   a. The adult and child within the family;
   b. The adult in the workplace and the child in school;
   c. The social lives of both adult and child;

4. The family's adaptation to the disease.

THE PARENT

Extent of the Disease and Its Complications

The 22 parents we interviewed ranged in age from 28 to 72. The average age of diagnosis for the parents in our study was 35. Of the 15 who had CMT, four were mildly affected, nine moderately affected, and two severely impaired. For the purposes of this study we defined "mildly" as appearing normal to others but having some disability, such as a person with hand involvement who has trouble with fine motor tasks, or a person who has high arches and is beginning to have foot and balance problems. "Moderately" we defined as having had surgery, or needing braces or orthopedic shoes. Such a person might have trouble walking, especially on uneven surfaces, or using stairs. "Severely" disabled was defined as being confined to a wheelchair or motorized scooter.

Many people with CMT, even those with braces and canes, look and act very normal. This normal appearance is one of the reasons physicians (and others) tend to dismiss their complaints. Most of the parents in our survey were active, involved, and working. However 13 of the 15 affected parents reported that having CMT limited what they could do. They reported that at times they felt anger, frustration, and depression because of these restrictions. They also experienced these feelings when physicians dismissed their problems. Several said that their disease proved to be an embarrassment when they were not able to do everyday things.

How Does CMT Affect Performance in the Family?

Parents felt that they were often limited in the types of things they could do with their families. The restrictions parents experienced ranged from being unable to handle routine tasks to not being able to participate in activities that unaffected families take for granted. Curbs, stairs, hills, and having to walk long distances presented obstacles that required planning . . . or avoidance. Many found that the steep steps and lack of hand rails in theaters and stadiums made it difficult to attend cultural or sports events.

When balance was affected, carrying a child, using a ladder, walking up and down stairs, carrying groceries, or even taking out the garbage presented problems. For those with hand involvement, there was often loss of feeling, and tasks involving fine motor coordination could be difficult. Several people told of needing help cutting meat, or buttoning or zipping clothing.

In the Workplace

Here too, activities that unaffected people take for granted, such as business travel, routine office tasks, taking care of small children, or standing at a lectern to deliver a speech or teach a class, presented problems. A person whose job required travel found managing suitcases—both carrying them and lifting them on or off the conveyer belts at airports—very difficult. The manager of the parts department of an auto dealership said that because of a lack of feeling, papers and pencils often slipped from his hands. He had to concentrate to keep this from happening as he dealt with customers and supplies.

In all, nine of the parents said that their CMT created difficulties for them at work.

Socially

The same restrictions that limited people within the family and workplace also limited people socially. Those who were severely affected found that needing a wheelchair or motorized vehicle prevented them from visiting friends, attending church functions, or even going to the post office or bank. Several people mentioned that no longer being able to dance was emotionally painful and so they avoided events where dancing was a major part of the activities. Several reported that dating was awkward. Someone who has a strange gait or needs braces or a cane often does not find it easy to get dates. As anthropologist R. F. Murphy points out, "Whatever the physically impaired person may think of himself, he is attributed a negative identity by society, and much of his social life is a struggle against this imposed image" (1987, p. 113). Also the reality of the disease limits where one can go or what one can do on a date. Three people said that fatigue limited their social lives and two people said that they had become more introverted because of having CMT. On the other hand, a woman who is severely impaired and confined to a wheelchair reports that she has a very active social life. She has just made arrangements to go ballooning.

THE CHILD

Extent of the Disease and Its Complications

In the 22 families we interviewed, there were 27 children who had CMT. Their ages ranged from 3½ to 52. Eleven children were mildly impaired (four females; seven males). One of these children had a mild scoliosis. We included her because there appears to be a relationship between scoliosis and CMT (NFPMA, 1988, p. 16). Eight had moderate involvement (five females; three males). Six were severely impaired (three females; three males). Two who had been diagnosed exhibited no symptoms. Three families had two children with the disease and one family had three children with it.

Performance in the Family

Children who have neuromuscular diseases often have special needs and these needs can place a strain on family members. There are often frequent doctor visits, sometimes a need for corrective surgery and/or physical therapy. Depending on the degree of impairment, young children often needed help putting on braces, dressing, or eating. Parents reported that when a child had corrective surgery, the long recovery period was taxing on the entire family. They found this time to be physically, emotionally, and in some instances financially draining. One mother with a master's degree told of having to give up her teaching job because the school would not give her a long enough leave of absence to take care of her postoperative child. She lost income, seniority, and tenure. Parents of twelve of the children reported that their children needed some special attention.

Parents also reported that their children with CMT were physically unable to keep up with siblings, both younger and older. Some found that children became annoyed or frustrated when they could not do what other children did or had to depend on others to do things for them. The fatigue and lack of stamina that adults described also seemed to be a problem for children. Three parents said that their affected children had periods of being moody and withdrawn. But, as one parent pointed out, "We tend to blame a lot on CMT; whether or not the kids' moods are connected to their having the disease, who knows?"

In School

Ten children had problems in school. Some of these problems were directly related to the attitudes of school personnel, who often treated children with physical disabilities as though they also had intellectual impairments. One of the complaints parents had was that often their children with CMT were not encouraged or helped to catch up on missed schoolwork. A severely impaired child whose IQ was near genius level was not challenged because her teachers refused to see her physical disability as just that . . . a physical problem.

The parent of a 25-year-old reported that being in a wheelchair prevented her son from attending classes that were above the first floor. The school made no allowances for his condition and when he didn't get to class, no one was concerned.

Some of the problems were related to the attitudes of other children. Even a mild case of CMT can limit what a child can do, especially in sports and gym. Several children told their parents that when this happened, the kids made fun of them. Two parents reported that they still experience pain when they think of the cruel remarks they heard as children. One said that because of her strange gait, the kids used to call her ducky. Another told of kids who used to walk behind her and quack. Even those who have received special attention feel a stigma. One little girl who was a Muscular Dystrophy Association poster child alternated between showing off her braces and feeling upset because she was different from other kids.

Socially

Only six parents said that the disease interfered with their children's social lives. Those who seemed to be having the most problems, as expected, were those who were severely impaired. They often could not participate in normal children's activities, and the same social, emotional, and physical barriers that exist for adults also exist for children. Making friends was difficult since other children usually do not reach out to those with disabilities. As one mother of a severely impaired child said, "Children are often afraid to approach a child with a handicap." Another parent put it a little differently: "It takes a special person to befriend a severely impaired child."

CONCERNS OF PARENTS

We also asked parents what worried them most about CMT. Because of the uncertainty of the progression of the disease, and society's attitude towards those with disabilities, a major concern was what would happen to their children. Only two said that they were not worried. A number of parents said that they also worried about their own future.

IMPACT ON THE FAMILY

Barbara Sabbeth, in her article, "Understanding The Impact of Chronic Childhood Illness On Families" (1984, p. 55), has stated, "The impact of an illness from the parents' point of view is often surprisingly different from the impact from the physician's point of view. To add to the complexity, the impact of the disease on the mother from the mother's point of view (that is, according to her self-report) may be different from the impact on the mother from the point of view of an observer." We asked the parents to rate how stressful CMT has been on their families. We gave them a scale from one to five with one being little or no impact and five being severe. Two parents rated it a one. Five parents said that they would give it a two and five parents a three. Two said it was a four. Six parents rated it a five and found it extremely stressful. Two parents refused to answer.

Of the six parents who found it extremely stressful, three did not have the disease themselves. Of the other three, two were moderately affected and one had it severely. The parent who had it severely also had a child with severe involvement.

ENCOURAGING CHILDREN
TO DEVELOP OTHER ABILITIES

Seventeen parents said that they had encouraged their children to develop in ways that did not require physical stamina. This encouragement took many forms. Some helped their children to develop intellectually; some involved their preschoolers in arts and crafts so that they would not feel compelled to get into sports as they got older. One parent arranged for her daughter to have voice lessons. Others, while making their children aware that they might have some limitations, encouraged them to do whatever they wanted.

THOUGHTS OF NOT HAVING CHILDREN
OR LIMITING THE FAMILY

As we stated in the introduction, the average age of diagnosis for the parents was 35. Eleven of the parents had children by the time they found out that they had CMT. Two had grandchildren. Several were diagnosed only after their children had been diagnosed. A number of adults said that if they had known they had an hereditary disease they might not have had children. Four parents decided not to have any more children after their children were diagnosed. One man and two women were aware that they carried an hereditary disease and still decided to have children. However they said that they were not informed that it was possible to have a child more severely impaired than they. Also neither woman realized that CMT might worsen with pregnancy. Both women reported that pregnancy had not only exacerbated their disease but they also had children with severe involvement and suffer enormous guilt. One woman had asked her physician about the risks of having children. He brushed off her concern by saying: "What's the problem? You can still walk."

The idea of passing down a genetic defect also seemed to produce guilt in parents. Thirteen parents, not all of whom had CMT, reported this. Two parents, because of the guilt and suffering they experienced, had even suggested that their children seriously consider not having children and had encouraged them to seek genetic counseling.

EXPENSES

A family that has a member with a chronic medical condition, such as CMT, can have many expenses. Depending on the severity of the disease, there can be a need for extra medical care or special equipment such as braces, canes, orthopedic shoes, or a wheelchair. The Muscular Dystrophy Association will provide care and its physicians are familiar with CMT. They will also pick up many expenses. However people with CMT are not always referred to them.

Sometimes there are less obvious expenses such as a need for household help or a need to make changes to accommodate a worsening of the disease. One parent, who could no longer manage stairs, told of having to move from a two-story house to a ranch; another had to equip her house with ramps.

RELATIONSHIP WITH SPOUSE

Six spouses said that the disease affected their relationships but in a positive way; they became closer. Nine said that it had a negative effect. Two husbands left because they could not handle their children's illnesses.

TALKING ABOUT CMT WITHIN THE FAMILY

Three parents reported that they did not talk about it in their families and said that their spouses were not open to discussing it. For most, this was not an issue and it was talked about openly.

LACK OF INFORMATION ABOUT CMT

Over three quarters of the parents said that the lack of information about Charcot-Marie-Tooth disease was stressful. Forty percent found it very stressful.

FEELINGS OF LOSS

We all go through life with expectations . . . expectations for what we will do, become, or have. These expectations are not just for ourselves but also include those closest to us. Some of these expectations are realistic; some are not. When a member of a family has an illness such as CMT, many hopes can be shattered and there is a sense of loss or a need to mourn for what he or she no longer has or may never have. Those who can no longer dance and find it difficult going to events where dancing is a major part of the activities are feeling this loss. Every member of a family in which there is an illness such as CMT has to deal with it. The person who is no longer able to work, the father whose son will never become an athlete, the mother whose daughter will never become a surgeon, or the child whose brother or sister is unable to take part in children's games, all experience loss.

Fifteen of the parents said that they experience feelings of loss and a need to mourn, especially for their children.

Sometimes this feeling of loss takes the form of denial. It can be seen in the parents who push their children into various endeavors, especially athletics. Two parents report that this is an issue in their families. It seems that they hope involving their children in sports will either ward off the disease or prove that their children do not have it. Both these families also have problems talking about CMT.

FAMILY ADJUSTMENT TO CMT

Almost 60 percent felt that they had adjusted. In the two families where a parent was severely impaired, one parent said that she had adjusted. The woman who had not, had a severely impaired son, and her husband had left the family.

Of the other families who had a child with severe CMT, three said that they had adjusted. However, one of these was a parent who would not rate the impact of CMT on the family.

DISCUSSION

This is not an in-depth study and our sample is small. What this study does is look at a rare disease within the context of the individual, the family, and society and give an idea of what it is like to have CMT. It speaks about relationships — relationships between an individual and his or her disease, relationships between the individual and family, and relationships between the individual and society. But within these relationships are the seeds for research. This preliminary study raises many questions that are worthy of investigation.

CMT, while it can restrict what one can do, and while it can be extremely incapacitating, did not affect all the respondents in the same way. Also, the degree of impairment seemed to have little to do with how limiting people found it or how well they said they had adjusted.

A person's personality, attitude about illness, and perception of loss of integrity all play a role in how well he or she copes or adjusts. Perhaps the extrovert has an easier time of it than the introvert.

Family attitudes about disease and disability are also important. Sabbeth argues, "Each family has its own mythology, which is passed from one generation to the next, thus linking the family to its past and contributing to the creation of its future. Family myths, based on fact as well as on fiction, include attitudes toward birth, growth, sickness, and death; they shape and are shaped by the serious illness of a child" (1984, p. 55). What happens to a child whose family remains in denial for a period of years or a child whose family cannot come to terms with his or her disability? What message does the child get about himself or herself and how does this affect him or her in adulthood?

Are families in which a parent has CMT different from those in which a parent does not have the disease? It seems that they might be. Parents who have CMT seem to find it less stressful and seem to "adjust" more easily than parents who do not. Interestingly, all of the seven parents who do not have the disease have encouraged their children to develop talents and interests that do not require physical ability.

Society's attitudes also play a role in how well a person handles his or her disease. How much does the stigma our society attaches to having a disability affect a person with CMT (see Goffman, 1986)? What is it like for a person with CMT to experience social and physical barriers? How do the cruel comments of classmates or the prejudice of school personnel affect a person with CMT?

A better-informed medical community could make a difference as far as diagnosing and referring, although it seems that this is beginning to happen. The children in the study were diagnosed at a younger age than the parents. However, this could be because they had a more severe form of CMT than the older respondents. A more empathetic medical community could also make a difference.

Finally, what is it like knowing that one has a hereditary disease of which there is little awareness and which generates little research? We need research into the causes of CMT and we need to know that people are working on cures. We also need to know how the disease affects both individuals and families as we realize that it will be a long time before medical research provides us with any answers. It is the hope of the authors of this preliminary study that it will serve to stimulate this very necessary research.

REFERENCES

Cassell, E. J. 1982. "The Nature of Suffering and the Goals of Medicine." *The New England Journal of Medicine* 306:639-645.

Goffman, E. 1963. *Stigma*. New York: Simon and Schuster, Inc.

Leventhal, J. M. 1984. "Psychosocial Assessment of Children with Chronic Physical Disease." *Pediatric Clinics of North America* 31(1):71-86.

Murphy, R. F. 1987. *The Body Silent*. New York: Henry Holt and Company.

National Fund for Peroneal Muscular Atrophy. 1987. *NFPMA Report* 1(1).

National Fund for Peroneal Muscular Atrophy. 1988. *NFPMA Report* 2(2).

Sabbeth, B. 1984. "Understanding the Impact of Chronic Childhood Illness on Families." *Pediatric Clinics of North America* 31(1):47-57.

ADDITIONAL READING

Bateson, G. 1972. *Steps to an Ecology of Mind*. New York: Ballantine Books.

Bateson, G. 1980. *Mind and Nature*. New York: Bantam Books.

Bateson, G. and M. C. Bateson. 1984. *Angels Fear: Towards an Epistemology of the Sacred*. New York: Macmillan.

Buchanan, D. C. 1979. "Reactions of Families to Children with Duchenne Muscular Dystrophy." *General Hospital Psychiatry* 1:262-269.

Gayton, W. F. 1977. "Children with Cystic Fibrosis: Psychological Test Findings, Siblings and Parents." *Pediatrics* 59:888-894.

Holyroyd, J. and Guthrie, D. 1986. "Family Stress with Chronic Childhood Illness." *Journal of Clinical Psychology* 42:552-561.

Matthews, L. and D. Drotar. 1984. "Cystic Fibrosis: A Challenging Long-Term Disease." *Pediatric Clinics of North America* 31:133-151.

Perrin, E. C. and P. S. Gerrity, 1984. "Development of Children with a Chronic Illness." *Pediatric Clinics of North America* 31:19-31.

Perrin, J. M. and H. T. Ireys. 1984. "The Organization of Services for Chronically Ill Children and Their Families." *Pediatric Clinics of North America* 31:235-257.

Travis, G. 1976. *Development of Children with a Chronic Illness*. Stanford, CT: Stanford University Press.

Helping Patients Cope with Acute Loss of Neuromuscular Function

Ramaswamy Viswanathan

In the game of chess, the Queen is the most important piece (besides the King) for a very obvious reason: it has the maximum range and direction of movement, which give it great power. Movement is very important for a person's mental and physical health. A patient with neuromuscular dysfunction finds not only that his physical health is impaired, but that his coping options are also restricted because his movement or communicating ability is impaired. The therapeutic challenge is to help the patient feel as much like a "Queen" as possible by maximizing movement through rehabilitation and modern technology, and also to help the patient realize that even if much movement is not possible, he is still a "King" for his family and friends.

In this article the focus will be on acute onset of dysfunction in adult life. (Childhood onset of dysfunction has additional effects by its impact upon physical and psychological development processes.) I will discuss how patients can be helped to cope with acute loss of neuromuscular function, and present some case examples from my experience as a psychiatric consultant to medical and surgical inpatient services.

STRESSORS ASSOCIATED
WITH NEUROMUSCULAR DYSFUNCTION

The psychological and physical benefits of movement and the dangers of inactivity are well known. The so-called "jogging mania" that is sweeping the world is due to the perceived physical benefits as well as the "runner's high." Movement also gives us greater control over our envi-

Ramaswamy Viswanathan, MD, is Clinical Associate Professor of Psychiatry and Associate Director of Psychiatric Consultation—Liaison Service, State University of New York Health Science Center at Brooklyn, 450 Clarkson Avenue, Box 127, Brooklyn, NY 11203.

155

ronment, facilitates social interaction, and increases recreational opportunities. Modern devices such as automobiles and planes have extended our mobility. We have been so accustomed to this expanded range of movement that many of us feel "down" even if our car is temporarily disabled or our flight is delayed. One can imagine the depression and frustration of those who lose control over their own bodies.

Depending on the site and degree of neuromuscular dysfunction experienced by the patient, and his or her personality and life situation, a patient may experience one or more of the following stressors:

Loss of sense of control: We have a need to feel in control of our body and our environment (Beiber 1980). When this is threatened or lost, severe emotional distress and a sense of helplessness, anxiety, and depression may ensue (Viswanathan and Vizner 1984; Viswanathan and Kachur 1986).

Loss of sense of integrity: We have a sense of "wholeness" of body and mind. Dysfunction threatens this sense of integrity.

Dependency on others: The idea of being dependent on others is disturbing to many. Many experience guilt or shame. This may lead to low self-esteem, and may interfere with the patient communicating his needs and getting proper help. When one is dependent on others for basic biological needs such as elimination and eating, the sense of inadequacy and helplessness can be especially strong.

Frustration: When one is dependent on another, there is a delay between one's thought and the action of the other that can be frustrating. A common complaint that the author hears from many patients is that others (nurses, doctors, family) do not respond fast enough or do not respond at all. This is especially distressing when bladder or bowel needs or pain relief are not attended to immediately. There is also the problem that the other may not perceive one's needs correctly.

Cosmetic losses: This can be due to not being able to look after one's appearance properly, or factors such as disuse atrophy or contractures.

Changes in one's social status and role, and support system: One may find that one does not have as much power and authority as before, or that people do not associate with one as much as they used to.

Financial losses.

Inactivity and boredom.

Limitation of coping options: Inability to move around decreases the range of coping activities one can engage in.

Loss of dignity and quality of life.

Threat to life or threat of further deterioration in health: This may be due to underlying disease process or greater susceptibility to infections and thromboembolic complications.

HOW PATIENTS CAN BE HELPED TO COPE

An understanding of the nature of coping mechanisms is useful in devising ways to help a patient cope with the trauma of neuromuscular dysfunction. Coping can be broadly divided into instrumental and palliative coping mechanisms (Monat and Lazarus 1977). Instrumental coping involves taking action to change the situation. Palliative coping involves changing one's perception of the situation. (It is analogous to obtaining pain relief by taking an analgesic medication.) Both kinds of coping are required in most cases. It is important to help patients develop a "coping orientation" instead of just feeling helpless.

Instrumental Coping

Whenever possible, instrumental coping should be encouraged. This could be physiotherapy to increase the strength and range of movement, learning new ways of doing things, making use of tools such as wheelchairs and various assist devices, and of course trying to correct the underlying problem (e.g., taking anticholinesterase agents to relieve the symptoms of myasthenia gravis).

Palliative Coping

When the dysfunction cannot be corrected totally, one has to be able to accept the loss and live with the dysfunction. Even when total recovery of function is possible, palliative coping is still needed to reduce emotional distress during the recovery process. In many instances palliative coping reduces emotional distress and helps the individual concentrate his or her energies on instrumental coping. In some instances, some kinds of palliative coping can be maladaptive by interfering with instrumental coping. For example, a person with a transient ischemic attack of the brain who uses denial ("everything is fine") to cope with the condition may not seek medical help. The following are some examples of palliative coping:

Buying time: In my inpatient consultation work I find this a very valuable approach when I am called to see patients with acute loss of function who are very demoralized and do not have any concept of rehabilitation. Such patients have to be helped to maintain hope and patience. Educating them about rehabilitation, asking them to wait for a specified period of time to see how things work out, and pointing out that they always have the option of withdrawing from treatment later often remarkably improve their mood and willingness to engage in treatment. One is making no false promises, one is merely asking these patients to subject themselves to life experiences for a period of time to develop a more realistic perspective on their problems. It also gives time for healing and coping mechanisms to evolve, and gives time for psychotherapeutic interventions.

Hope: Hope is very important to coping and treatment, and also to reducing emotional distress. One has to encourage hope, taking care to see that the expectations are realistic, in order to avoid the negative effects of later disappointments. Seeing or learning about others who have recovered from or coped successfully with similar problems can be enormously helpful. Religious patients should be encouraged to make use of their religious faith.

Finding meaning and purpose in life and in what has happened: Frankl (1963), the founder of logotherapy, found that finding meaning and purpose in one's life was helpful in coping with catastrophic experiences such as concentration camps. I have found this to be a very important principle in helping patients who have severe illnesses and suffer serious losses. Many find meaning in living for their family. Some engage in helping others overcome similar distress or help others in need. Some lead extremely productive lives despite handicaps. In the acute situation, all these avenues have to be pointed out to the patient. Finding meaning and purpose in what has happened is harder. But many religions teach this. When patients are religious and take the view that God must have had some purpose in making it happen, even though the purpose is not always apparent to us mortals, it reduces their distress.

Changing internal dialogue, relabeling or reinterpreting the situation, and selective attention: The Greek philosopher Epictetus remarked: "Men are disturbed not by things but by the views which they take of them" (cited in Beck et al. 1979). Cognitive therapists have pointed out that what we pay attention to and what we tell ourselves about a situation affect our mood, that we have control over our emotions, and that we can change our emotions by changing our internal dialogue — our thinking about the situation (Beck et al. 1979; Meichenbaum 1977). For example, if a patient is saying to himself "No, I am not helpless; there are things I can do to improve the situation; let me see what I can do." If he has the thought, "Everybody rejects me," he can be asked to examine this idea carefully; he may discover that while some do reject him, there are still others who do love and accept him, and that in some situations he is misinterpreting certain behaviors as rejections because of his sensitivity. In this instance he may change his internal dialogue to, "It is unfortunate that some people reject me; but I am happy that there are still others who love me and accept me; let me concentrate my attention on these people."

Distraction: This is a type of selective attention, in which one is totally removing attention from a particular idea. Examples are watching television, reading a book, or chatting with others. One problem with the hospital situation is that it is difficult to distract oneself, to keep one's mind occupied much of the time. Occupational therapy is important in the rehabilitation process, as being meaningfully and creatively occupied is an effective distractor. Altruistic behaviors (helping others) are also effective distractors. Of course, both of these have the important benefits of promoting self-esteem and sense of purpose, adequacy, utility, and acceptance.

Relaxation: Apart from reducing anxiety and tension, relaxation also improves the patient's sense of being in control.

Psychotropic medication: In some situations psychotropic medications may be called for as adjuncts to psychological treatment. If a patient develops major depression, he will need antidepressants in addition to psychotherapy. If there is excessive anxiety, he may benefit by use of anxiolytics as adjuncts to psychological intervention.

Obviously the social support system is important for both kinds of coping. The patient has to experience respect and love of others. Family support increases the patient's sense of security. Family intervention is important to help the family cope with the stress of the patient's illness and to promote optimal interactions between the patient and the family. For example, the family has to be helped to promote the patient's independence and offer needed support at the same time.

CASE ILLUSTRATIONS

Diana

Diana was a 35-year-old woman with a renal transplant who suddenly developed left hemiparesis, visual impairment, and rejection of the transplanted kidney, all due to multiple arterial emboli. When I saw her initially, she was (understandably) very apprehensive about the sudden and progressive loss of various functions. She needed administration of antianxiety medication (intramuscular injections of lorazepam) to control her severe anxiety. Later she became profoundly withdrawn and depressed, did not want to live anymore, and refused all treatment. She saw life as useless, felt that she was a burden on her husband, and felt hopeless. She had no will to live. Quick exploration with her husband in her presence demonstrated to her that she was still very valuable to her husband. She was asked to find a purpose to live for. She decided that her purpose in life was to live for her family. But she was distraught by her neuromuscular dysfunction and felt this would not improve. This was one reason she felt like refusing all treatment, including dialysis, and "ending it all." I told her that I understood her feelings, and that many people feel like this in the acute stage, as it is hard for them to appreciate the potential for rehabilitation, and as they have not had sufficient time to develop ways of coping with their losses; that many are later surprised to find how, with rehabilitation, medical efforts, and the passage of time, they are able to function much better. I told her that perhaps she could give herself a few weeks to experience the recovery process. If she still felt like stopping dialysis and other treatment, and giving up, she could do that. She was agreeable to this therapeutic trial.

A few days after beginning physical therapy, Diana began crying and became depressed because her husband was indicating that she was not working hard enough in rehabilitation and did not appreciate her limitations due to pain. This matter was explored with her husband in her presence; it was pointed out to him that it was common for many spouses to be well-meaning but to put too much pressure on the patient, and that it could have the opposite effect, increasing the patient's sense of inadequacy and alienating her from him when she needed the husband's closeness the most. The husband understood it and the patient also saw (relabeled) her husband's behavior as well-intentioned. Spousal relationship became much better after this. The patient engaged energetically in the rehabilitation program and her mood and physical functioning improved remarkably over the next few weeks.

John

John was a 68-year-old widower with squamous cell carcinoma of the hypopharynx, treated with radiotherapy and chemotherapy, who developed difficulty in walking due to muscle weakness (cancer-associated myopathy), and difficulty in swallowing. He appeared depressed and had significant psychomotor retardation. He had insomnia and very poor appetite. Nursing staff described him as just lying in bed all day long, not doing anything, and not engaging in conversation. He was started on desipramine and began responding. He expressed severe depressive ideation because of his inability to walk. "What good am I if I am not able to get around?" he said. He was unable even to get out of bed on his own. He felt life was not worth living and had thoughts of jumping out the window.

I recommended to the oncologist that promptly initiating rehabilitation was very important to this patient's emotional recovery. Initially John was not interested in rehabilitation as he felt that he would never be able to walk again. But he agreed to "give it a try" after he was given an explanation about the rehabilitation process with some examples, and asked to give himself a trial experience for a few weeks. After he started physical therapy, in the beginning he felt it was too tiring and wanted to give up. I taught him to say to himself, "I should view the muscle tiredness as a sign that I have had a good workout. Even though it is unpleasant, I will bear it as it will help me to walk." While he began improving physically, he still tended to focus on the fact that he was unable to walk, and he continued to feel dejected. He was asked to pay attention to the progress he was making and remind himself that this was a sign that he was progressing toward the goal of walking. This helped him to persist in physical therapy. His physical strength and mood gradually improved. One day he was able to get out of bed, walk to the bathroom, and pass urine unassisted. He was very excited about this accomplishment. He continued to improve. He did not have suicidal ideation anymore. His interest in life and relationships returned.

Joe

Joe was a 35-year-old man with end-stage renal disease who had become acutely depressed following rejection of his transplanted kidney (donated by his father). He refused hemodialysis because he saw life on hemodialysis as not worth living, because he believed that it would interfere with his career plans. After psychotherapeutic intervention, he changed his mind and decided to try hemodialysis for a period of time. Several months later, after receiving training for home hemodialysis, he began developing slurring of speech and weakness of legs on the day his home-dialysis equipment was to arrive at his home. His physician initially thought that it might be a conversion reaction. I felt that it was likely to be a neurological problem, probably a polyneuritis. He turned out to have Guillain-Barre syndrome.

Joe became depressed because of his difficulty in communicating and because he had become dependent on others for many things. His father spent most of the day by this bedside helping him. Joe experienced considerable rage toward his father, feeling that his father did not understand or respect his feelings in many matters. Psychotherapy focused on his guilt at the loss of his father's kidney and its intensification by his enforced dependency on his father again, as well as the disease's interference with his life plans. A couple of conjoint sessions focusing on the father-son interactions relating to his dependency were also helpful. The patient experienced considerable anxiety because of his neurological impairments, especially at night when he was left alone. It responded to relaxation training, supportive psychotherapy, and the antianxiety medication buspirone (which was chosen in this instance because, unlike benzodiazepines, it is not a respiratory depressant). When physical therapy was begun, the patient became demoralized at his weakness, tiredness, and "slow" progress. This was dealt with by asking him to be patient, to focus his attention on acknowledging to himself the progress he has made so far, and to remind himself that this was evidence that he was progressing toward full recovery of his physical function. The patient was able to leave the hospital with substantial improvements in his physical status and mood.

Sam

Sam, a 40-year-old man with amyotrophic lateral sclerosis, was refusing many blood tests. His house physicians interpreted this behavior as "depression" and requested psychiatric consultation to evaluate whether the patient could benefit by antidepressant medication. The patient was not ambulatory, was on a respirator, and had a Foley's urethral catheter. Even though he could not vocalize, the nursing staff could understand his speech by observing his lips. I was impressed by the attention and care many nurses were giving him. Even nurses who were not taking care of him on a particular day would chat with him and spend time with him. The nursing staff did not see any problematic depression on the part of the patient and felt that he was coping adequately with his situation. The patient's wife visited him daily and spent considerable time with him. She fed him lunch and dinner daily and he ate well.

I interviewed Sam with the help of a nurse serving as interpreter of his lip movements. The patient was grateful that his wife and the nurses were so kind to him and spent so much time with him. He acknowledged that he had a terrible illness and indicated that he was using his faith in God and prayer to help him cope. He was satisfied that everything possible was being done for his care. He said that he refused many blood tests as he did not see any point in doing them. I pointed out to the house staff that this patient was coping quite well, was interacting with wife and staff to the best of his ability, and was not rejecting food offered by his wife; that his refusal of many tests was not a manifestation of clinical depression but an understandable response, since from his point of view they were not going to be of significant help to him; and that there was certainly no indication for antidepressant medication. Further explorations brought out the fact that the house staff experienced discomfort in taking care of a young, alert person who was definitely terminally ill and whom they could not cure; the tests gave them a feeling of doing something "concrete," and when they were refused by the patient, antidepressant medication was viewed as another concrete thing to do. I pointed out to the house staff that the patient was already getting the most important intervention, namely care and attention from his wife and several nurses, and he seemed to be pleased with it. The major things they could do would be to show interest in him as a person, to not avoid him because of their discomfort about being unable to offer him hope for a cure, and to reduce his suffering to the extent possible.

As the cases demonstrate, acute loss of neuromuscular function can be emotionally devastating. Where partial or complete recovery of function is possible, the health care team and the family can play an important role in helping the patient cope with the losses and focus on rehabilitation and recovery. Even when no hope for improvement is possible, they can still help the patient by demonstrating to the patient that he is still valuable as a person.

REFERENCES

Beck, A. T., A. J. Rush, B. F. Shaw, and G. Emery. 1979. *Cognitive Therapy of Depression*. New York: Guilford.

Beiber, I. 1980. *Cognitive Psychoanalysis*. New York: Jason Aronson.

Frankl, V. E. 1963. *Man's Search for Meaning*. New York: Pocket Books.

Meichenbaum, D. *Cognitive-Behavior Modification*. New York: Plenum.

Monat, A. and Lazarus, R. 1977. "Stress and Coping: Some Current Issues and Controversies." In A. Monat and R. Lazarus, eds., *Stress and Coping*. New York: Columbia University Press, pp. 1-11.

Viswanathan, R. and E. K. Kachur. 1986. "Development of Agoraphobia After Surviving Cancer." *General Hospital Psychiatry* 8:127-132.

Viswanathan, R. and T. Vizner. 1984. "The Experience of Myocardial Infarction as a Threat to One's Personal Adequacy." *General Hospital Psychiatry* 6:83-89.

Grief Management by Spouses
of Neuromuscular Disease Patients

Peggy Reubens

Much has been said about bereavement after a death. This essay discusses the losses suffered by spouses of neuromuscular patients during the lives of these patients. For the purpose of this paper, "spouses" includes all committed partners, regardless of gender or legal sanction, as well as ex-spouses who get reinvolved in end-stage caregiving.

It may be underrecognized that spouses of all chronically ill patients grieve significant losses even before death threatens. What is different about neuromuscular disease is its assault on the very sense of self, as the abilities to move and communicate are challenged. The social being is equally challenged, and it is this social being that is married to someone. In diseases that remit, such as multiple sclerosis or myasthenia gravis, or that vary daily, such as Parkinson's, the social roles are uneasy and future planning may suffer. In the progressive atrophies, there is a steady erosion of the social self, with increasing dependence on family. When these patients are married, their spouses not only bear extra burdens but also feel losses. These losses may be overlooked as family discussions focus on financial and work-load stresses.

The periodic or progressive losses sustained by a partner are experienced differently by different individuals, and may be denied or displaced onto concrete concerns. But there is a grieving process, however covert and unsanctioned it may be. Even conflicted relationships meet many critical human needs, including the need for assistance, for reassurance of worth, for nurturance of shared goals, and for some degree of intimacy, if only via shared history.

Yet the attention of health care staff, family, and friends is so focused on the devastation suffered by the patient that the spouse's losses may be

Peggy Reubens, ACSW, is former Supervisor of the Department of Social Work Services, Neurological Institute, New York, NY, and is in private practice at 60 Riverside Drive, New York, NY 10024.

overlooked. The spouse who voices grief may be accused of self-centeredness or it may be suggested that he or she has a psychiatric problem. No matter if the spouse is experiencing anticipatory grief at the time of first diagnosis, grief at an exacerbation, or mourning at the end-stage, many staff have little time or tolerance for these partners who seem self-involved or self-pitying. Social workers, while trained to empathize, may appear heartless to spouses; they are pressured to make discharge plans at a time when family grieving mitigates against the clear thinking needed for that planning.

Even when among other spouses in support groups, many partners censor their own expression of grief. They either deny any emotion or are only able to describe anger, never sadness. Helping professionals need to validate the expressions of grief that do emerge, as well as to help those in denial to contact their sadness and express it.

In a review of the literature on illness and the family, very little seemed to address the grief of the spouse or partner. There is literature on the family's effect on the patient, or the effect of a child's chronic illness on the parents, but not on the effect of an adult's illness on the spouse. It may be that the family studies field has to "catch up with" the number of chronically ill adults medical technology is now able to keep alive and at home so much longer than before. With the neuromuscular diseases, there is a critical need to develop such understanding.

VARIATIONS IN GRIEF MANAGEMENT

Gender

In general, women in our culture are more sanctioned to grieve and to discuss feelings than are men. In addition, there may be more of a loss for wives than husbands of neuromuscular patients: the protective aspect of the male role is reinforced by a wife's incapacity, while the incapacity of a husband is felt as a major loss to older women who are used to being protected. As more couples engage in equalitarian relationships, this may shift. It is still too easy to label a grieving wife helpless and dependent, instead of identifying her grief.

Age and Relationship Duration

Some older spouses may be more accepting of loss; others grieve as acutely as younger people. The diseases discussed here largely affect young to middle-aged adults, and thus emotional and sexual losses may be far-ranging. Interruption of goals also occurs, and may include cancellation of child-bearing plans, loss of coparenting functions, and reduction of lifestyle goals. Professionals need to help these spouses mourn their specific losses, before they can be helped to revise goals and develop substitute support systems and activities.

Meaning of Loss to Spouse

To help the spouse move on, we must discover the meaning of his or her loss, including prior experience with grieving.

A 30-year-old woman had suffered no major losses prior to her husband's acute onset of multiple sclerosis. She had no experience with grief management for her loss of companionship, which she expressed as, "He's just not the same person I married." For several years, she seemed stuck in either depression or rage at her husband or helpers. This situation improved when it was found that her grief related to her position in her family, one in which she felt she wasn't allowed to have or keep anything important.

A 45-year-old husband of a mid-stage, hospitalized amyotrophic lateral sclerosis patient grieved both for his wife and for himself (with some encouragement). The son of two Holocaust survivors, one of whom died of cancer in the man's teen years, this man had grown up steeped in defenses against overwhelming grief. He seemed to need no professional intervention until his wife's discharge home approached. Suddenly, no respirator would satisfy him; all home health aides were inadequate and possibly larcenous. The obstacles to taking his wife home multiplied daily. Ultimately, pressed by the social worker, he broke down and sobbed, "When I take her home it's always like the start of a new nightmare."

For other spouses, the experience with grieving has been tempered by years spent with illness. Some have suggested that spouses pass through stages that parallel Kübler-Ross's schema for patients. Others feel these stages apply less broadly. The wife of a Friedreich's ataxia patient described herself as hopeful for a cure after years spent in disbelief, then anger and fear, then hopeless depression, alternating with guilty feelings about resenting her husband and shameful feelings about wanting to hide him from public view. Few husbands of neuromuscular patients evince similar guilt or shame. Some admit to depression; many skip from anger directly to a type of acceptance, if not actually hope.

Culture

Traditional family units that have an expectation that "life is hard" bolster spouses in group grieving and other customs and rituals for grief. Grief seems more accessible as there is less shock and disbelief that such a tragedy can happen; religious faith provides a route to acceptance. The ability to believe in a divine plan helps make sense out of losses, which is a key technique in grief management.

Time and Space

Does the spouse have space to grieve or is he or she totally absorbed in attending to the grieving patient?

Does the spouse have time to grieve, amid caregiver tasks, employment, children and other demands? Reality and the defensive use of reality can combine so that the partner exhibits stress but not grief.

The most overt grieving may be seen in spouses of less needy patients, who are also more comfortable financially. This does not mean that the financially stressed spouses described above are not grieving or that professionals should not try to help that emotion surface. Of course, if the partner needs to hold on to denial, that should be respected as a tool of grief management.

Individual Coping Styles

Of course, spouses may have developed individual coping styles to deal with previous losses and disappointments. These may include: anger, major depressions, self-absorption, distractions, focus on concrete issues, search for miracle cures, substitute relationships, infidelity, development of their own physical symptoms, or a philosophical or religious acceptance of fate. In stable and remitting situations, the partner may adapt to the needs the patient can still meet and hopefully view the patient as more than a body or its symptoms. Partners of progressively ill people may have to accept cumulative losses until reaching a symbolic "death" that they mourn before biological death occurs.

However, when coping styles seem problematic, it is important to assess the couple's functioning as a system.

THE COUPLE AS A SYSTEM

It is arguably true that much dysfunctional couple behavior relating to illness stems from unrecognized, unsanctioned, incomplete, or warded-off grieving. Given time, energy, and insight, individuals may work these things through. But in many situations, a systems intervention with the couple is more practical.

A noted family therapist, Jerry M. Lewis, has written that "most models of the impact of stress on the family do not attend sufficiently to the role of the family's pre-stress organization and structure as a significant determinant of the outcome" (Lewis 1979, p. 104). In his model, pre-stress styles of couple interaction can predict styles that will ensue from severe or chronic stress.

Distance regulation is a central dynamic for all couples. Early in the relationship, couples have to deal with commitment, intimacy, and power issues, and each of these dimensions can be seen to determine the degree of closeness or distance between them, as well as how stable or fluctuating that distance will be over time. What Lewis types as healthy couples develop flexible family systems that contain both closeness and bounded separateness. For these spouses, grief management may depend on revaluing or prioritizing the basic relational needs to fit current circumstances.

Some goals may have to be altered; much physical assistance is no longer possible; some forms of intimacy need to change—but emotional intimacy, reassurance, and nurturance are still possible because the patient is not overly self-absorbed, and the spouse is not overly merged, in these couple systems. These are also the spouses who seem able to develop substitute supports while the patient is still alive.

But under prolonged stress, even close and flexible couples may develop a more distant and rigid style in order to cope. In Lewis' terms, their style would become dominant-submissive, in which power is no longer shared and intimacy is limited.

After many years of illness, the neuromuscular patient may take on a submissive role, due to dependence on the spouse. Mr. M, an ALS patient, became tyrannical with his wife, even when his speech could no longer be his vehicle. Mrs. M was helped to recognize that beneath her husband's rage was a massive fear of submission. Under that was enormous grief for the lost days of equality.

The Js, on the other hand, were a couple who agreed that Mr. J had always been the "boss." Mrs. J had rapidly progressing MS and expressed gratitude for having a "strong man" while she grew weaker. Some years later, when she became wheelchair-bound, this couple seemed to have progressed to what Lewis terms the conflicted style. Mr. J criticized his wife's needs and she seemed to unwittingly thwart him with the timing of those needs, specifically, her incontinence. In therapy, Mr. J was restored to an empowered position once he confronted and grieved for his wife's loss of bladder control.

Lewis postulates that couples whose style has been conflicted (in their pre-stress life together) will become chaotic under severe or chronic stress conditions. Chaotic couples have few boundaries between them and tend to merge, but so fear the environment that they cling together, albeit in an ineffective way. They may remain so through the course of the illness; the well spouse may flee, or with help, such couples can reorganize.

Knowing these concepts of couple organization can help professionals to assist clients to their optimum level of functioning even under the stress of neuromuscular disease.

REFERENCE

Lewis, J. M. 1979. *How's Your Family?* New York: Brunner-Mazel.

Whose Hell is Hotter—
Yours or Mine?

Ed Gallagher

Whose hell is hotter—
Yours or mine?
No, I don't know
how or what you feel
I can only guess—ONLY guess
And that's all
you can do with me

Whose hell is hotter—
Yours or mine?
I'm sure we'll agree
it viciously attacks
in varying degrees
and brutally burns
when . . . WE LET IT

Whose hell is hotter—
Yours or mine?
Cool faces mask ferocious fires
Don't go by mine
I don't go by yours

Whose hell is hotter—
Yours or mine?
My crippled body
doesn't mean
I have it worse than you!

Ed Gallagher is Independent Scholar, Foundation of Thanatology, New York, NY, and is Writer, Producer, and Host, Cable Access Commission, White Plains, NY.

Be with me, friend
I'll be with you
Let's water ourselves
with candid conversation

I MAY get a clue
and so MIGHT you
from one . . . blazing question

Whose hell is hotter —
yours or mine?

SECTION II: CLINICAL AND RESEARCH CONSIDERATIONS

Rehabilitation Concerns in Late-Stage, Ventilator-Dependent Muscular Dystrophy Patients

Agatha P. Colbert
Francis J. Curran

The increasing use of ventilators in patients with Duchenne muscular dystrophy (DMD) (Alexander et al. 1979; Curran 1981; Bach et al. 1981; Rideau et al. 1983; Colbert and Schock 1985) has resulted in a growing population of individuals with advanced muscle disease who are living well beyond the expected second decade. The decision to extend life in a young person with a rapidly progressive neuromuscular disease is a complex one for all concerned. Difficulties are multiplied as a consequence of the absence of long-term followup data. The quality of life extension and the associated medical, rehabilitative and psychosocial concerns in DMD are unique because of the age group involved and the progressive nature of the disease. Although a few studies have assessed quality of survival for individuals with DMD (Gilgoff 1983; Snyder and Goldberg 1983; Miller,

Agatha P. Colbert, MD, is Director, MDA Clinic, and is Consultant Psychiatrist, Lakeville Hospital, Lakeville, MA 02347. Francis J. Curran, MD, is Director of the Pulmonary Department at Lakeville Hospital.

Colbert, and Schock 1988) there remains relatively little published on the natural history of the disease in persons with DMD who choose to use supportive ventilation.

Over the past ten years, through the New England Medical Center and Lakeville Hospital Muscular Dystrophy Association clinics, we have been involved in the care of 30 patients with DMD, using ventilators. This article attempts to summarize our clinical experience.

Our DMD patients developed respiratory failure at an average age of 19.8 years (12.8 to 29.1 years). Their mean long-term survival since initiation of ventilatory assistance has been 5.4 years (0.4 to 12.3 years) (see Table 1). Seven of the 30 have died.

Six of the 23 survivors live independently in their own apartments and rely on personal care attendants for their daily living needs: six reside in their parental homes utilizing personal care attendants as primary caregivers and family members as backup: four live with their parents and depend on them for their total care: five others are in a chronic care hospital: the remaining two attend a state hospital school during the week and are home with their families on weekends. Only one individual in this group is married; he has two children, aged five and two years. Eight have participated in higher education or have completed a college degree. None are gainfully employed at this time.

Seven patients are deceased, having used the ventilator for periods of three months to six years. Although the clinical circumstances surrounding the terminal event were apparent in all, the precise cause of death remains undocumented since no autopsies were performed. Four were found dead at home in their functioning ventilators; two of this group had been recovering from a flu-like syndrome; the other two had no intercurrent illnesses and were apparently in their usual state of health. Three patients died in the hospital, one of cardiac failure after a stormy and protracted course in the intensive care unit. Another expired as a result of an acute cardiorespiratory crisis from which he could not be resuscitated; the seventh patient, from complications of severe obstipation with abdominal distention and secondary diaphragmatic elevation. His death occurred during an attempted intubation. It appears that most patients have died as a result of primary or secondary cardiac complications, but more data needs to be obtained on causes of death and manner of dying. In cases of rapid demise we suspect a cardiac dysrhythmia as the most probable cause of death, but this needs to be looked at in more depth. Many parents and individuals deciding to accept assisted ventilation are seeking information about the circumstances attending death if a ventilator is used. Our experience to date in this area is limited.

ONSET OF RESPIRATORY FAILURE

The vast majority of patients (25) presented with symptoms of chronic respiratory insufficiency rather than acute respiratory failure. The most frequently observed symptoms were: morning headache; disruption of sleep patterns, i.e., wakefulness and restlessness at night and daytime drowsiness; weight loss; daytime dysphoria; and fatigue. Families described several weeks to months of a nightmarish time prior to the diagnosis of respiratory failure during which they found it impossible to make their child completely comfortable. For them the decision to accept ventilatory support was made because it offered immediate relief of symptoms rather than because it meant an extended life expectancy.

Of the five patients presenting with acute medical emergencies, one had a mixed clinical picture of combined cardiorespiratory embarrassment and four had primarily respiratory compromise. All of these required immediate admission to the hospital and intensive intervention. The others were diagnosed with chronic respiratory failure, recognized during a routine clinic visit. We might mention that it took a few years of clinical experience to be able to differentiate the symptoms of respiratory failure such as headache, sleep disturbances, or a general lack of thriving from other conditions, especially depression. We found, however, that these symptoms were remarkably consistent and corroborated with abnormal arterial blood gases when chronic restrictive pulmonary disease was present.

The medical parameters heralding the onset of respiratory failure in the 30 patients included a progressive decrease in vital capacity to an average of 498 mls (15% of predicted) and an average elevation of pCO_2 to 60 mm Hg (see Table 1).

When patients were diagnosed with chronic respiratory failure they were admitted to the hospital for a two- to three-week trial of different ventilators. The appropriate ventilator was one which could be tolerated by the individual and was effective in ventilating him through the night. The table also lists the initial ventilators used and the supplementary aids provided over the subsequent years. A comprehensive description of these devices is provided in an article by Hill (1986).

Negative pressure systems were more frequently utilized because of availability, patient preference, and physician bias. The practice advocated by staff at Lakeville Hospital and NEMC as well as by Aberion et al. (1973), Alexander et al. (1979), Bach et al. (1981) and Hill (1986) is to offer a noninvasive form of ventilation to persons with restrictive lung disease whenever possible. When pulmonary compromise is a result of a progressive neuromuscular disorder, the onset of respiratory failure is

TABLE 1. Patient Data

Subject	Onset Type	Age Onset (Years)	pCO2 mmHG	VC (mls)	Years of use	Devices
SD*	chronic	12.8	62	–	0.8	Iron lung
CB	chronic	15.1	50	336	5.3	Iron lung
DR	chronic	15.4	55	470	3.2	Iron lung
EA	chronic	16.5	51	445	6.2	Iron lung & MIPPV
WM	acute	16.5	70	580	3.5	Iron lung
MP	acute	16.9	70	–	10.8	Trach & PPV
KC	chronic	17.0	54	357	7.9	Cuirass: Iron lung & pneumobelt
SA*	chronic	17.0	56	930	2.0	Poncho wrap
JD*	acute	17.1	–	1200	0.4	Trach & PPV
RM	chronic	17.6	59	432	8.2	Iron lung
LT	chronic	17.9	56	500	5.6	Trocki vent: iron lung MIPPV
JH	chronic	18.0	81	303	2.0	Iron lung
EO	chronic	18.1	48	700	4.2	Iron lung
WM	chronic	18.8	53	546	4.0	Iron lung
PR	chronic	18.9	49	600	4.7	Poncho wrap:iron lung & MIPPV
JH+	chronic	19.0	49	280	6.1	Iron lung & MIPPV
MD	chronic	19.5	60	302	12.3	Iron lung & MIPPV
KF	chronic	19.8	68	400	9.1	Iron lung & MIPPV

CS*	chronic	20.2	51	432	1.2	Iron lung
GR	chronic	20.7	44	618	5.2	Iron lung & MIPPV
SC	chronic	21.1	56	376	8.4	Trocki vent:iron lung & MIPPV
SD	chronic	21.9	63	486	7.5	Iron lung & MIPPV
MD	chronic	22.3	54	450	8.4	Iron lung:trach & PPV
TA*	chronic	23.4	80	-	1.3	Iron lung
RC	acute	23.5	78	388	11.7	Iron lung
MC	chronic	24.0	64	350	5.1	Pneumobelt:trach & PPV
WR	chronic	25.0	66	460	3.5	Iron lung
KM*	chronic	25.1	51	504	4.1	Iron lung
TS	chronic	27.5	88	900	5.7	Iron lung & pneumobelt
MG	acute	29.1	-	-	3.3	Trach & PPV
Averages		19.8	60	498	5.4	

*Deceased

Key: MIPPV   = mouth intermittent positive pressure ventilator
Trach and PPV = tracheostomy and positive pressure ventilator
Trocki vent = customized body ventilator

slow and the initial need for supportive ventilation is usually only during nighttime hours (Curran 1981). In the early stages of chronic respiratory failure, body ventilators have been found to be satisfactory for most individuals. As more hours on the machine are required however, alternate devices with or without a tracheostomy were implemented.

The choice of an individual's ventilator was made on the basis of its efficiency of ventilation, and patient comfort and convenience. The physiological goal for satisfactory use of a device was to decrease the pCO2 to below 40 mm Hg while in the ventilator and to have it remain below 50 mm Hg after five or more hours of independence from the ventilator during the day.

Twenty-seven patients required ventilatory assistance at night only for the first two to three years of use. A small minority, three patients, required 24-hour-per-day ventilation at the onset. Two presented with acute pneumonia requiring full-time assistance with a tracheostomy and positive pressure ventilation for a period of three months at which time they were weaned to nighttime use only. They have continued to be ventilated with a positive pressure device through the tracheostomy. The other, a 17-year-old, presented in cardiorespiratory failure and was admitted to the intensive care unit when he was intubated. Over the subsequent five months he suffered a left-sided cardiovascular accident, leaving him aphasic, and severe congestive heart failure, which was aggressively treated, according to his mother's wishes. He was not unlike the case described by Snyder and Goldberg (1983) who spent the last and most painful months of his life in the intensive care unit.

CLINICAL COURSE

Over the years, as the respiratory muscles become weaker, patients have been obliged to increase their number of hours of assisted ventilation. The clinical indications for more time on the ventilator were evidenced by a recurrence of symptoms of hypercapnea (carbon dioxide retention) and the increased dependence of glossopharyngeal breathing (frog breathing) in many. One young man developed a mycoplasma pneumonia and could no longer be supported with his pneumobelt. Although the iron lung was adequate for his ventilation, he felt it limited his mobility and therefore restricted his lifestyle excessively. As a consequence he opted for a tracheostomy with positive pressure. The physical findings in the others correlated with a progressive decline in vital capacity at a rate of 42 cc per year and a gradually rising pCO2 level after being out of the ventilator for a few hours.

OTHER MEDICAL COMPLICATIONS

The provision of a mechanical ventilator helps to circumvent respiratory failure and prolongs life but does not seem to influence the course of the disease in any other way. Progressive symptomatology experienced by the majority of this patient population included problems with organ systems such as the gastrointestinal, respiratory, cardiac, and musculoskeletal.

Gastrointestinal

Seventy to 80% of patients complained of gastrointestinal symptoms such as difficulty chewing and/or swallowing, constipation, abdominal discomfort, and weight loss. The chewing and swallowing problems seem to be the result of progressive weakness and contractures of the masseter and pharyngeal muscles. Three patients have had a gastrostomy tube inserted with a resultant weight gain. These individuals continue to be fed orally as well as through their G-tubes. Constipation is a major concern in 82% and, as noted above, led to death in one case.

Respiratory

Respiratory complaints included frequent colds, congestion, fatigue, and the returning symptoms of hypercapnea. Shortness of breath was a problem for 82%. A persistent problem with a few patients has been the acute and very frightening experience of what they call "congestion." This appears to be caused by mucus caught in the trachea which cannot be dislodged because of inability to cough vigorously—a situation that is particularly aggravated when the individual is seated. During such an occurrence, patients describe a sense of panic and a feeling that they must be returned to their ventilators in order to be assisted in moving the mucus plug. Attempts to move the mucus with high pressure on an intermittent positive pressure system have been ineffective and the "Coughlator," which was commonly used in the polio era, is no longer commercially available. The etiology of this "congestion" is unclear. In some cases it began with a bout of bronchitis but persisted several months after the infection had resolved. With a few patients this problem has resulted in a life confined to immediate home environs. An alternative approach for these people might be a tracheostomy to allow emergency suctioning and permit continued mobility, if that is desired.

With progression of respiratory muscle weakness into daytime chronic respiratory failure, patients using negative pressure ventilators or devices that work optimally in the supine position were severely limited in their mobility. At the present time we are trying alternative, noninvasive, portable ventilators. Several patients are utilizing mouth intermittent positive pressure ventilators (MIPPV) with the sippy pipe or the Bennett lipseal. Bach and Alba (personal communication) employ MIPPV as the treatment of choice in their patient populations. Recently nasal positive pressure has gained wider acceptance in clinical practice (Bach et al. 1987; DiMarco et al. 1987) and may prove to be an acceptable positive pressure alternative to other negative pressure body ventilators.

Cardiac

Cardiac symptomatology has been less clearly defined than the respiratory complaints. All persons with DMD have a degree of cardiomyopathy. It is uncertain why some develop more cardiac than respiratory problems as their primary presentation. There is generally less stress placed on the heart muscle because of an individual's extremely impaired motoric ability throughout the course of the disease. In the advanced stages of DMD, echocardiograms show very little compensatory cardiac reserve, and it seems quite likely that stresses such as an infection or an episode of severe constipation could result in overwhelming cardiac failure or a fatal dysrhythmia.

We have not found electrocardiograms to be especially helpful in management, but serial chest x-rays to detect cardiac enlargement and echocardiograms have been beneficial in defining those patients at greatest risk of becoming symptomatic. Although there are few treatment possibilities for severe cardiomyopathy, this knowledge will provide the patient and his family more information on the overall prognosis and possible cause of death. Tachycardias, including paroxysmal atrial tachycardia (PAT), are treated with calcium channel blockers such as verapamil, which effectively reduces the heart rate and is specific for reentry types of arrhythmias.

Musculoskeletal

Progressive musculoskeletal weakness, deformity, and discomfort was seen in all patients. Those who had no previous spinal fusion, with the exception of one 12-year-old boy, have scoliotic curves of at least 35 degrees. In addition, we have witnessed further scoliosis progression after age 20 years, even in those persons with "fixed, extended spines" as described by Gibson (1978). Back discomfort as well as impaired respiratory effort compel many of the patients to adopt a semireclined position in their wheelchairs. Physiologically this permits less crowding of the diaphragm and eases the respiratory effort. However this position further reduces their functional abilities and creates the need for technically complex wheelchair controls and customized seating and mobility systems.

In the advanced stages of DMD, further weakness and contractures develop in the neck, trunk, and upper extremities, leading to additional functional impairment. At the onset of respiratory failure all of our patients had enough upper extremity strength to drive their motorized wheelchairs with hand-controlled joysticks. They continued to do so for three to five years. However, in the ensuing years, the majority of patients have had to resort to use of a very sensitive, short throw, hand-operated joystick or a chin or tongue type of control as the result of weakness.

FUNCTIONAL CONSIDERATIONS
IN SEATING AND MOBILITY

Throughout the course of DMD, patients seem to define for themselves a critical point of balance to compensate for weakness and to enhance function. They achieve this by means of certain well-recognized movement patterns. During the ambulatory phase, these children develop a means of weight shifting that allows them to maintain the center of gravity behind the hips and in front of the knees. This is accomplished by assuming an excessively lordotic lumbar posture and by rising up on their toes. In the wheelchair stage of the disease a similar precarious point of balance is sought in order to maximize upper extremity function. Many individuals with DMD will sit far forward in the wheelchair with a similar lordosis and use their head position rather than their weakened upper extremities to balance themselves. Interestingly, we have noted that following spinal fusion many boys lose functional abilities such as the capacity to feed themselves because of their mechanically restricted back mobility. Prior to surgery they may have lacked the necessary shoulder and elbow flexor strength to bring the hand to the mouth but were able to compensate by bringing their mouths to their hands. This feat is no longer possible following spinal stabilization.

As functional skills become more limited, the main goal of the rehabilitation team is to help maintain an optimal quality of life by providing appropriate technological aids to maximize independent mobility and function while assuring comfort and efficient ventilation.

When prescribing a motorized wheelchair for a 16 or 17 year old with DMD, the anticipated progressive impairment and associated needs of the next 5 to 10 years must be taken into consideration. If the individual has decided to accept a ventilatory aid when that becomes necessary, a special customized frame and a ventilator tray will be an essential part of the wheelchair prescription. In addition, a power reclining mechanism should be included to permit independent position changes and relief of pressure areas as well as to enhance respiratory effort in the semireclined posture. We have observed that an extremely sensitive joystick will be necessary at some time for all patients with DMD but it may be counterproductive to supply this too early on. This type of control may be easily damaged if operated by moderately strong hand and forearm muscles. Consequently one must be certain that the chair prescribed is compatible with the type of joystick that may be necessary in the future.

Contoured seating systems are often necessary in order to offer support and comfort in the presence of musculoskeletal deformities. We have had reasonable success with custom-molded orthotic devices such as the DE-SEMO seat, the Contour-U system, and the Mold and Hold MacLaren seat.

CONCLUSION

Over the past 10 years of participating in the care of young men with DMD, considerable insight has been gained with regard to the long-term morbidity and mortality for those individuals choosing to prolong life with artificial ventilators. The progressive course of the disease is essentially unaltered but the quality of survival can certainly be enhanced by the early and aggressive prevention of contractures and spinal deformities, the assiduous monitoring of pulmonary function, attention to general health and nutritional aspects, and the provision of appropriate durable medical equipment. The decision to ventilate someone with a rapidly progressive neuromuscular disease is wrought with medical and ethical dilemmas. We hope this paper contributes to enhancing the knowledge of anticipated medical problems in advanced DMD, and assists patients, families and medical professionals in making an informed choice about ventilator use.

REFERENCES

Aberion, G., A. Alba, M. H. Lee, and M. Solomon. 1973. "Pulmonary Care of Duchenne Type Muscular Dystrophy." *New York State Journal of Medicine* 15:1206-1207.

Alexander, M. A., E. W. Johnson, J. Petty, and D. Stauch. 1979. "Mechanical Ventilation in Patients with Late Stage Muscular Dystrophy: Management in the Home." *Archives of Physical Medicine and Rehabilitation* 60:289-292.

Bach, J., A. Alba, L. A. Pilkington, and M. Lee. 1981. "Long-Term Rehabilitation in Advanced Stage of Childhood Onset Rapidly Progressive Muscular Dystrophy." *Archives of Physical Medicine and Rehabilitation* 62:328-331.

Bach, J. R., A. Alba, R. Mosher, and A. Delaubier. 1987. "Intermittent Positive Pressure Ventilation via Nasal Access in the Management of Respiratory Insufficiency." *Chest* 92:168-170.

Bach, J. R., A. S. Alba, G. Bohatiuk, L. Saporito, and M. Lee. 1987. "Mouth Intermittent Positive Pressure Ventilation in the Management of Post-polio Respiratory Insufficiency." *Chest* 91:859-864.

Colbert, A. P., and N. C. Schock. 1985. "Respirator Use in Progressive Neuromuscular Diseases." *Archives of Physical Medicine and Rehabilitation* 66:760-762.

Curran, F. J. 1981. "Night Ventilation in Body Respirators for Patients with Chronic Respiratory Failure Due to Late Stage Duchenne Muscular Dystrophy." *Archives of Physical Medicine and Rehabilitation* 62:270-274.

DiMarco, A. F., A. E. Connors, M. D. Altose. 1987. "Management of Chronic Alveolar Hypoventilation with Nasal Positive Pressure Breathing." *Chest* 92:952-954.

Gibson, D. A., J. Koreska, D. Robertson, A. Kahn III, and A. M. Albisser. 1978. "Management of Spinal Deformity in Duchenne Muscular Dystrophy." *Orthopedic Clinics of North America* 9:437-450.

Gilgoff, I. S. 1983. "End Stage Duchenne Patients: Choosing Between Respiratory and Natural Death." In L. I. Charash, S. G. Wolf, A. H. Kutscher, R. E. Lovelace, and M. S. Hale, eds. *Psychosocial Aspects of Muscular Dystrophy and Allied Diseases: Commitment to Life, Health, and Function*. Springfield, IL: Charles C Thomas, p. 301-307.

Hill, N. 1986. "Clinical Applications of Body Ventilators." *Chest* 90:897-905.

Rideau, Y., G. Gatin, J. Bach, and G. Gines. 1983. "Prolongation of Life in Duchenne's Muscular Dystrophy." *Acta Neurologica* 5:118-124.

Miller, J. R., A. P. Colbert, and N. C. Schock. 1988. "Ventilator Use in Progressive Neuromuscular Disease: Impact on Patients and Families." *Developmental Medicine and Child Neurology* 30(2):200-207.

Snyder, R. D. and N. M. Goldberg. 1983. "Use of Ventilator Support in the Terminal Care of Duchenne Muscular Dystrophy." In L. I. Charash, S. G. Wolf, A. H. Kutscher, R. E. Lovelace, and M. S. Hale, eds. *Psychosocial Aspects of Muscular Dystrophy and Allied Diseases: Commitment to Life, Health, and Function*. Springfield, IL: Charles C Thomas, pp. 41-44.

The Ventilator Support of Patients with Neuromuscular Disorders

Colin D. Hall
James F. Howard, Jr.
James F. Donohue

For most patients with progressive neuromuscular disease, the complication which is likely to lead to death is respiratory failure due to fatigue of the respiratory muscles. Technological advances in pulmonary care have given us the ability to support failing respiratory muscles and therefore prolong life in a significant number of these patients. This will generally involve the use of some form of mechanical ventilation. In acute and reversible disease, this is clearly of major benefit and rarely presents ethical problems for the patient, the family, or the caregivers. With chronic and protracted disease, the decision to intervene is much more difficult for all involved. Aside from the question of whether respiratory support is medically feasible, there are major practical and ethical issues that must be addressed. Generally, patients and their families have no background knowledge or experience on which they can base a decision to accept or reject mechanical ventilation. They must depend on the advice of the health profession.

The practical questions that must be answered relate to which type of ventilation will be most beneficial, when ventilatory assistance is required, where the ventilator-supported patient will live, and who will look after the patient and maintain the equipment. The ethical questions are really centered on quality of life issues. Will the patient on a ventilator be able to enjoy life enough that it is a reasonable alternative to death? In this article, we would like to share our recent experience with patients who

Colin D. Hall, MB, ChB, is Director, Neuromuscular Unit and Professor of Neurology and Medicine, University of North Carolina School of Medicine, Chapel Hill, NC 27514. James F. Howard, Jr., MD, and James F. Donohue, MD, are affiliated with the Departments of Neurology and Medicine, University of North Carolina School of Medicine.

have been followed at the Neuromuscular Clinic at the University of North Carolina at Chapel Hill, and who have elected to accept ventilator support for their chronic progressive neuromuscular disease.

Our overriding philosophy is that we, as the medical team, have primary responsibility for diagnosis, for deciding if a patient has reached the stage at which ventilatory support is necessary to sustain life, and for deciding if it is technically feasible for an individual patient to be successfully ventilated. However, we do not, and should not, make the decision as to whether the person will actually be ventilated. This decision must be made by the patient, with the help of those close to him or her. Although this may sound obvious, we are very conscious of the fact that our influence could be unduly obtrusive, and we must be very careful not to instill unwarranted optimism, pessimism, or guilt in patients and families. We have a responsibility to impart accurate information in a way that can be easily understood, and clearly this entails that we ourselves understand the circumstances that dictate whether ventilation is or is not successful.

To help understand these circumstances, we have evaluated the course of illness in the last 17 patients who elected to use mechanical ventilation and made a decision as to whether this treatment could be regarded as successful or not. We based our decision on information from three different sources: the patient's interpretation as to whether the quality of life had been sufficient to say that extension of life had been worthwhile, the family's impression, and our own medical team's interpretation of the effects on all involved. We understand that this is a rather crude method for coming to such a weighted conclusion, but in fact the answer was usually quite obvious for each given patient. We then tried to correlate the quality of life in each patient with a series of variables, to see if we could identify factors that were likely to predict a successful or unsuccessful outcome.

First, we will describe briefly our strategy for presenting the options to the families. Table 1 lists the various members of the team involved in this presentation, and any or all of them may spend time in discussion with the family before the decision is made. Each has his or her own particular expertise and viewpoint to contribute.

An early decision is when the topic should be broached to the patient and family. This will depend to some extent on the disease process, but we have a general policy with the flexibility to adapt it for the individual. The possibility of ventilatory support is discussed whenever the patient initiates the topic. Otherwise, if the patient does not require respiratory assistance but there is a likelihood he or she may already have been concerned about respiratory failure "down the road," initial fleeting refer-

TABLE 1

TEAM INVOLVED IN TRAINING AND EQUIPPING PATIENT

NEUROMUSCULAR SPECIALIST
PULMONOLOGIST
NEUROMUSCULAR NURSE
PULMONARY NURSE
PULMONARY FUNCTION LABORATORY
RESPIRATORY THERAPIST
SOCIAL WORKER
EQUIPMENT PROVIDER
OTORHINOLARYNGOLOGIST (Tracheostomy)

ence is made as reassurance, letting the patient know that there are ways to prevent inability to breathe "if the worst should occur," and if that is his or her wish. We also reassure the patient about feeding by use of a gastrostomy if that seems appropriate.

As respiratory difficulties develop, the possibilities are fully discussed with the patient and family in the clinic, and this is reinforced by a letter of explanation. This letter is very helpful in avoiding the misinterpretation of information given in the stressful setting of the clinic. It also allows the patient to share information with others who were not present for the conference. We have also arranged access to other respirator-dependent patients and their families, to try to give families a better impression of what is involved in the decision.

This is a crucial point in the decision-making process. We have found it less traumatic for patients to elect *not* to be ventilated than for them to ask for the ventilator to be turned off once they are established on it. However, despite our best efforts, the true magnitude of the decision is difficult to impart. We have been told by most families after the event that the rigors of care for the ventilated patient and the disruption of the household cannot be really understood in advance. Families at this stage also have to face considerable guilt—the patient for putting this burden on the rest of the family, and the rest of the family for their negative feelings about the demands on them.

If the decision is taken to accept ventilation, the patient is admitted to the hospital for training. We have found it is virtually impossible to obtain nursing home beds for ventilated patients, and so it is understood from the outset that the object is to return the patient to his or her home with whatever nursing support is available, but with family members playing a major role in caregiving. During the hospitalization, ventilation is started, and the family is trained in its use. The family is instructed in use of the machine, suctioning, and tracheal toilet. These techniques are demonstrated, and then the family is observed performing them, to ensure that they have fully understood the process. This is accompanied by a written explanation of all material covered and a written evaluation and checklist for the family's use.

We have used only two types of ventilation, a negative pressure cuirass and a positive pressure ventilator. We have found that a nasal positive pressure mask and the use of rocker beds have been inadequate for the needs of these patients in anything but the short term. The cuirass has several advantages: it is easily and noninvasively fitted, often not requiring a tracheostomy; for those who do not require continuous support it allows easy intermittent use; it is more comfortable; there is greater patient control; there is no danger of hypocarbia from over ventilation; it is less costly to fit and maintain; it is easier to discontinue therapy if that decision is taken. Its disadvantages are that it is not suitable for patients with intrinsic lung disease, at times it cannot be used because of the misshapen chest walls of some neuromuscular patients, there is an increased risk of aspiration if the patient tries to eat while the negative pressure is working, and eventually it may not be powerful enough to allow adequate ventilation in the case of total respiratory muscle failure. In addition, negative pressure ventilators are not suitable in cases of upper airways obstruction.

The diagnosis for each of the 17 patients is shown in Table 2. We concluded that the ventilatory intervention could be regarded as successful in 11, unsuccessful in 4, and of questionable success in 2.

One patient aspirated orange juice and died while using a cuirass. In all other cases, success was determined not by the mechanics of intervention but by the psychosocial well-being of the patient and family. In one case, the mother was looked after by the daughter, who had to give up her job. This led to great strife between daughter and son-in-law, and the eventual dissolution of that already fragile marriage. In another, the patient was looked after by his wife. He remained fearful and angry, with great difficulty in losing control, and the unhappy situation persisted over a year, until his final death. The wife required psychiatric help. Another patient was placed on a positive pressure ventilator against her previously stated wishes, and before the team became involved in the case. She was looked after at home by her family for a short time, but persisted in her wishes to have no support, and the ventilator was switched off. An additional young patient was cared for at home for several months by a professional nursing service before death, as family and friends declined to play a role in his care. He expressed intense and continuous unhappiness, but declined to have ventilation discontinued.

Our conclusions as to what would indicate successful ventilatory intervention were limited by the numbers of patients involved. Our 4 failures were all in amyotrophic lateral sclerosis (ALS) patients, but 6 ALS patients were deemed to be successes. We concluded that the disease process did not determine the likelihood of successful intervention.

Eleven patients were on positive pressure machines from the onset, 5 were on cuirass ventilators throughout, and 1 patient switched from a cuirass to a positive pressure machine after some months. Eight successes were on positive pressure machines, 4 were on cuirass ventilators. We concluded that the type of ventilator did not significantly influence success.

TABLE 2

DIAGNOSIS IN VENTILATED PATIENTS

AMYOTROPHIC LATERAL SCLEROSIS	10
SPINAL MUSCULAR ATROPHY	2
MUSCULAR DSYTROPHY	3
DUCHENNE	1
BECKER	1
FACIOSCAPULOHUMERAL	1
CONGENITAL MYESTHENIA	1
POLYMYOSITIS	1
TOTAL	17

The ages of our successes ranged from 17 to 68 years, of our failures from 36 to 74 years. Age in itself did not preclude the likelihood of success, even in the elderly.

The time spent on the ventilator varied from 3 months to 6 years in the successes, from 1 month to two-and-a-half years in the failures. We feel that ventilatory intervention may be successful even if it is limited to only a few weeks. This may be enough to prepare the family better for the final event, to complete affairs which may be of extreme importance to the patient and to allow quality time for the patient in the terminal stages of their illness. Decisions should not be based solely on life expectancy.

We saw no clear relationship between the financial status of the family and the success of ventilation. It was clearly easier for more affluent families to obtain equipment and home help, but, with support from the medical team, adequate arrangements could be made, even for the impoverished.

Our experience has been that most cases of respiratory failure in neuromuscular disease can be technically successfully supported on artificial ventilation. We have concluded that 65% of our patients could be judged to have made the correct decision for them by electing to accept ventilatory support. This conclusion was reached by evaluating the quality of life of these patients and their families. Success was not determined by the diagnosis, the age of the patient, the length of time spent on the ventilator, financial status, or the type of ventilation used. The preexisting emotional strengths of the patient and family appeared to be paramount in a successful outcome. We also feel that careful and supportive presentation of the alternatives, at a timely interval before ventilation is required, is of great help to the families in making their choices. Careful family training on the use of equipment is of paramount importance for the physical and emotional success of treatment.

Our sample size is small, and we continue to evaluate our expanding experience in this group of patients.

A Note on Researcher Bias in Working with Terminally Ill Children

Richard A. Witte

Research on, as well as clinical work with, children with a progressive physical handicap that leads to early death is borne from, but also significantly influenced and limited by, the bias and emotions of the researcher. The researcher's anxieties, defenses, and guilt as they relate to the subject matter and subjects imperceptibly affect research methodology (both in setting up the project and in carrying it out) and interpretation of the information gathered. "Objectivity" is particularly stressed when the researcher *intimately* engages subjects and their stories. More vulnerable still to research bias is that researcher whose history includes unintegrated personal events of loss. Findings reported from such stressful research, then, are to some significant degree created, not just discovered, by the researcher.

When I first went to England eight years ago, I intended to work with a pediatric neurologist on a project involving leukemic children. This pediatrician originally contacted the University where I was to conduct my research at least six months before my arrival about setting up a play therapy project with leukemic children. The pediatrician broadly wanted to know what his child patients, who were facing a potentially terminal illness, thought and felt. The department knew of my interest in terminal illness through correspondence before I arrived. It was agreed that I would work in this area with this pediatrician.

After I arrived in England, it took over two months before the pediatrician and I sat down together over lunch to discuss the project. Once we did meet, I anticipated that we would discuss a research project that would include a fair number of leukemic children. Instead, his proposal was that I initially take one child in play therapy, and perhaps a few others would come my way if the play therapy with the first child worked well. We

---

Richard A. Witte, PhD, is Clinical Psychologist Director, Pacific Child and Family Guidance Center, and is also in private practice, Berkeley, CA.

concluded the lunch with a tour of the hospital and a promise that I would be contacted within a fortnight with the name of my first child. He never called, and I did not pursue him.

It is difficult to know exactly what went wrong with the beginnings of this project. From the time of his original interest, the pediatrician's enthusiasm diminished. I learned later from a child psychiatrist who had earlier worked with this man on a project with oncology nurses and parents of leukemic children, that the pediatrician, in her opinion a deeply empathic man, felt as his own the children's physical and psychological pain. She thought, therefore, that a close inspection of the children's affective responses to their deaths would have been extremely painful for him.

The pediatrician was not alone in his avoidance of the issue of death. Although I could defend myself with the rationalization of not wanting to be a "pushy" American when I first arrived to start this project, and although I made some attempts to expedite the launching of the project, I clearly did not force an earlier meeting. Doubtless, my decision to let him go was motivated both by my empathic understanding of his fears and by my lesser understanding of my own anxieties about confronting the issues of death and loss with children.

Next I was approached by an educational psychologist who worked in a neighboring educational authority. One of the schools he served was a physical handicap school, and in this particular school there were a number of children with Duchenne muscular dystrophy. He, as did the pediatrician earlier, envisioned a project with a limited play therapy offering. After I proposed a much larger research and clinical intervention project to include an expanded projective assessment, a psychodrama module, and extensive care staff and parent interviews, the educational psychologist pulled out his support. My suspicions as to the reason this man left the project after he proposed an intervention with dystrophic children were confirmed many months later when he confided that he did not think he could contend emotionally with the parents' tears over discussing their children's imminent deaths. This time, despite my equally intense fears, I lept blindly into a new course of inquiry.

I had the aid of an MA student at the University at the beginning of the project who helped me with some of the "sand tray worlds." About three weeks into this module, this student called me at home to inform me that one of the Duchenne boys, who was not in the research group, had died. He said that because of the death, he decided to stop making sand tray worlds with the children as he thought it was an invasion of their privacy.

Upon hearing the news, I went to the school to spend the evening with the children and care staff. No one talked about or even obliquely referred to the recent death. As a consequence of this experience, I decided that the projective test of making "worlds," rather than being an unwanted intrusion, could provide a way for the children to express their feelings about this ignored death. I spent the next day doing as many worlds with the children as I could. My formulation, of course, was that the student researcher had been no more exempt from anxiety about death than the rest of us, and his refusal to do the World Test around this emotionally tense time reflected his anxiety.

My supervisor and I talked on numerous occasions about the approach I would take in my intervention with the children, care staff, and parents on such sensitive subjects as early death and progressive disability. We agreed that with the children I would not directly broach the subject of death or disability, but would gather information on these issues indirectly through inference from the Make A World, Thematic Apperception Test, observation, interviews, and psychodrama. We enlisted the aid of an experienced psychodramatist. To bind our anxiety we carefully prepared each of eleven sessions, determining what areas *we* wanted the children to examine in the presence of the selected care-staff. The structure we imposed undoubtedly inhibited to some extent expression of the very feelings and ideas we hoped would emerge. I now strongly suspect that we unconsciously wanted to prevent, as strongly as we wanted to air, the emergence of some of this sensitive material. When the patients with dystrophies expressed fears of death and guilt over the extraordinary efforts their parents expended on their behalf, these issues came up as readily in discussion as drama work. In hindsight, the children, I feel, would have been more open to direct discussion about their fears than we previously thought was the case.

Similarly, with the parents and care-staff, we created a fairly structured interview schedule, but one which did not examine carefully or straightforwardly enough the effect of the disease on their personal emotional lives, including their private fears and grief. That is not to say that I did not get rich material from these interviews, but I could have gained richer material still had I been more direct in certain sensitive areas. When we created the interview schedules, we were unsure how the parents would receive a researcher (an American at that!) probing into their private lives. Our fears were that the caregivers would find me and my questions intrusive and disturbing. Nothing could have been further from the truth. In almost all cases, the parents welcomed, and in some instances, longed for, the opportunity to talk openly of their personal drama, triumph, and tragedy. Three examples follow.

My first interview was with Peter's mother. Two-thirds of the way through the interview I noted that the tape recorder had not been functioning for a half-hour. This mother suggested, at learning of *my* loss, that she be reinterviewed, this despite the fact that the interview was of such intensity that she and I could remember, close to verbatim, all the answers she had given in the previous 30 minutes as she talked about her son's impending death and disability. She was that invested in the task and that sensitive to my needs.

My second interview was with the parents of Andrew and Duncan. After a four-hour interview that culminated with tea and a debriefing, I had to break off the evening. The parents not only walked me to the door at 11:30 PM, but through their garden and down the road to my car. I had the fantasy that I could have taken them home with me that evening.

My last interview was an unplanned one. Another Duchenne boy, who once attended the school in which I conducted my research, died at age 18 years shortly before the end of my study. I was given the rare opportunity to interview the parents of this boy after his death. The mother generously granted me three hours of her evening. Upon my arrival the father offered me a gin and tonic, then left. Did he intend to address my anxieties or his own by his gracious offering? During the first part of the interview the father occasionally came in and out of the room, never staying for more than a moment; however, by the half-way point in the interview he was found sitting in the corner. By and by he offered a few observations and then took a great risk to talk poignantly about his private grief over losing his only son: the secret times he would cry alone after his wife went to bed; the need to be "strong" for his wife who carried the larger share of the physical caregiving efforts; the guilt he carried for maintaining an emotional distance from his son in an attempt to cope with his impending death. This mother was astonished by his admissions. They talked that evening for the first time since their son's diagnosis a dozen years earlier about the meanings it held for them.

I could go on with more examples, but suffice it to say, most of the parents were open to inquiry into very private material.

The eight months I spent collecting data on this project was not an easy time for me physically or emotionally. Besides conducting this research, I added to my schedule course work at the University and clinical work at the Child Guidance Clinic. However, simply citing this heavy schedule of my own creation does not fully convey the exhausting way in which the research was conducted at times. It was not only the numerous late evening interviews and observations that were physically numbing, but the emotional drain from immersing myself in the tragedy and pathos of the subjects' lives. I kept up a frantic pace, fearing that if I let up I would never return to the work. My activity level, at times, was nearly at a manic pace, and this description is not overstated for effect. There is no doubt in my mind that my frenetic activity kept depression at bay for me. On many occasions the death of my father, which occurred when I was an adolescent, emerged in my memory, as did my longing for my daughter who was separated from me for the year. Paradoxically, there were times when I found myself resenting my 7-year-old son, who was with me in England, and his dependency on me. I vividly recall one evening when I came back to the house after a cathartic psychodrama session in which one of the dystrophic boys, Calvin, broke down as he fearfully talked of his own death. Upon my arrival home, my son, Ben, bounded up to me with open arms, saying, "My dad's home." I coldly hugged him. My resentment toward him for being whole, without deformity, and with the prospect of a full life, unlike the dystrophic boy I just left, was so overwhelming at that moment that I actually had to send him away from me. I had lost my perspective on who Ben was for those few minutes as I was still depressively immersed in thoughts of Calvin. I had left the school that night, and other nights also, with feelings still engaged in deep sadness, desires to protect the children, and intense anger at the unfairness of the personal tragedy of their lives. There were moments, which I was only dimly aware of at the time, that afforded me experiential access to my subjects' feelings in a way that transcended my research data.

Yet it would be untruthful to say that this work was ultimately depressing. It had aspects of personal joy and intense gratification. There were moments I spent with these parents and adolescents in which the pretense of our respective roles and the distancing of our psychological defenses were stripped away. These were encounters which, I believe, affectively touched each of our lives. Certainly these times did so for me. In this work, I faced some of my own primitive fears and I survived, irreversibly changed in the encounter. Perhaps this is why I wished to work with death and dying in the first place. My perceptions of handicap and death have changed. As a result the confidence I have in myself and in the efficacy of my work have inexplicably increased in direct proportion to a growing understanding of limits to my knowledge and the acceptance on faith that what I am aiding in my psychotherapeutic work is a transformation beyond theory. My respect for the ability of the human spirit to love and live on despite the tragedy of the moment and of the future has been greatly deepened. My hope is that in some way my research has also given something of use to the children and to their parents.

Later, while I was struggling with the meaning of the research data and with writing it in narrative for my dissertation, my experiences were relived in my reverie nearly as intensely as when I was face-to-face with my subjects. It was exceedingly hard to leave this material. Although I had intended to finish writing the narrative on an up-beat note, I found myself writing an epilogue about the tragedy that the parents shortly still have to face. My chairperson convinced me not to include this chapter since the material contained in it was amply covered throughout the narrative. In the spirit of parallel process, perhaps I felt as the parents did that I was not doing enough, and to finish my writing felt like an abandonment of the children and parents. I left this dissertation enriched to go back into my vocation, a world that implies professional mobility and future. They, however, still have to finish the section I could delete.

Seated Thanks
to William Carlos Williams

Ed Gallagher

So
much
depends
upon
a
sturdy
wheelchair

K   I   S   S   E   D

with
morning
sunshine
beside
the
warm
bed

Ed Gallagher is Independent Scholar, Foundation of Thanatology, New York, NY, and is Writer, Producer, and Host, Cable Access Commission, White Plains, NY.

SECTION III:
IMPORTANCE OF SOCIAL SUPPORT

ALS Support Groups:
An Update

Claire F. Leach

Three years ago any of us working with groups of amyotrophic lateral sclerosis (ALS) patients did so mostly in isolation. This is no longer necessary with the evolution nationwide of an informal network that is both instructive and supportive. To further the exchange process among the proliferation of support groups, I undertook this survey to consolidate information about formats that have emerged and variable group elements about which choices are made regardless of format. I have sought the sponsors' own appraisal of their formats and found them almost universally satisfied that they are demonstrating their value and serving their purpose well. While the corollary is that some parts of the ALS population may not be attracted to and served by a particular format, it appears that all groups serve a substantial purpose.

The review is descriptive rather than statistical, discussing groups that are widely representative, with their variants. It is derived from my own valued personal contacts over the years; from additional interviews specifically for purposes of this paper with sponsors and moderators and with

Claire F. Leach, MSW, is Clinical Social Worker, Department of Neurology, Nassau County Medical Center, East Meadow, NY.

201

patient service coordinators in the national organizations, and from the very limited number of published articles about ALS support groups and interviews with their writers. Where an opinion or comparison or conclusion is mine, I have tried to identify it as such. The formulation of group types and contributing variables is mine. My perspective comes out of clinical social work training, counseling ALS patients and families in a neuromuscle clinic, moderating discussion and educational ALS support groups, and talking with many different moderators and sponsors. The material is to be looked at in the differing contexts of sponsorship, variable interrelated group components, and identifiable formats.

SPONSORSHIP

Groups usually represent one service of a local or regional ALS organization which has a number of other functions — research, fund-raising, public awareness activities, conferences, direct assistance, clinics, newsletters. They are presented under three principle auspices: the Muscular Dystrophy Association (MDA), the Amyotrophic Lateral Sclerosis Association (ALSA) and independent ALS centers and service organizations around the country.

In MDA, groups are actively and increasingly recommended by the national organization to its local offices as one of the most frequently sought and most effective means of helping neuromuscle patients and families. The impetus to start a group is usually from the local office of the countrywide paid MDA staff, often in conjunction with its 242 clinics, sometimes at the request of patients or caregivers. Format is often determined by a letter of inquiry to the ALS population registered with the local office. This gives considerable latitude to meet local needs and conditions. (A 10% response to a mailing is considered a good return.)

The two policy "givens" at the national level are professional leadership and a time-limited but renewable series. Facilitators are professionals with group training and/or experience and are paid by MDA unless group leadership is included in the clinic services for which MDA contracts. The time limit (6 to 8 weekly or biweekly sessions, 4 to 6 monthly sessions, or several planned quarterly sessions) exists in order to identify a point at which the program will be evaluated for future planning by the facilitator, MDA staff, and participants. In practice most meet monthly. Size is no less than five, for reasons of group process and economics, and preferably no more than 15 so that personal connections are encouraged. The group may consist of families only, patients only, or both, with patients-only groups being the rarest. ALS groups do not include people from any of the other disease categories covered by MDA because of the disease's unique demands on both patients and caregivers. They may present programs, exist primarily as discussion groups, undertake projects, or combine these approaches. Because of their number, a detailed canvass of MDA's clinics would shed valuable light on prevailing practice. Besides providing information one of MDA's stated primary purposes is to help ALS people realize they are not alone.

The variety of the ALS Association's group reflects that organization's less centralized relationship to its chapters and free-standing support groups. The chapters are locally autonomous and multifunctional, with varying histories and viewpoints. Some chapters directly sponsor groups led by psychiatrically-trained nurses and/or clinical social workers, usually on a monthly, continuous basis. Some chapters also guide and give support services to several small monthly groups in locations where people have requested them. To any such groups led by nonprofessionals, they supply local referral and resource information, administrative and moral support in terms of advice and literature, central informational meetings, and professional leadership if the group, the lay leader, or the chapter feels it would be useful.

Besides the 26 chapters, a number—currently over 75—of free-standing support groups have evolved in a kind of grassroots movement around the country. They originate typically with an inquiry to the national office with the goal of gaining information and emotional support. Most meet monthly, sometimes in people's homes. About a fifth are professionally moderated. Probably 90% are for patients and caregivers together. Some are philosophically committed to lay leadership by patient or family because personal experience with ALS is perceived as an essential source of understanding and support. Professionals attend these by invitation as specialists with a body of knowledge to impart. As the only groups I am aware of without the backing of a local ALS organization, the free-standing support groups look directly to the national ALS Association for support services and educational material, including guidance about coordinating a group. By affording this guidance, ALSA is helping to give form and direction to the urgency that is generated in patients and families who deal on a day-to-day basis with ALS.

Independent ALS centers comprise the third source of patterns for ALS groups. My contacts have been with those in San Francisco, Detroit, Chicago, Seattle, and Kansas, each with its distinctive parent organization and approach to support groups, each with its own highly distinctive character, philosophy, and flavor. All are creative, innovative, and continuing to develop. All are multifunctional and committed to groups as one essential element in a comprehensive approach to ALS. A description of the program of each one would be rewarding, but for present purposes I will extract the common features and highlight the unique ones from them and from the groups that have thrived within the national frameworks.

USING THE NETWORK

The independents and the national patient service offices of both MDA and ALSA have been generous with their time and thoughts and in their agreement to act as a resource to anyone wanting to consult them about their group management. Authors of the three published articles about ALS support groups and many sponsors and facilitators of groups across the country have been similarly responsive. Any may be approached by phone or letter. Addresses, phone numbers, and publishers are listed at the end of this paper as: Readings, National Organizations, and Sponsoring Organizations. The general type of group sponsored is indicated. Newsletters are also named. Taken together they are a gold mine of information, ideas, perspectives, and encouragement.

Information and insights about the status and dynamics of self-help groups and their relation to professionals is found in Thomas J. Powell's book *Self-Help Organizations and Professional Practice* (1986). Additional assistance to lay-led groups in developing goals, programs, strategies, leadership skills, and understanding of group process is available in the United States and Canada through national and regional offices of the Self-Help Clearinghouse.

CHOOSING THE VARIABLES

It is clear that the support group planners make choices about several of the same variables, whatever format results, and each choice tends to support a given emphasis in how to achieve group goals. All groups share at least implicit goals of comforting, sustaining, reinforcing positive defenses, teaching about the disease and practical coping techniques and resources, developing self-confidence and a sense of control, defining new hopes in the absence of cure, and putting ALS in its place within a meaningful life. All groups deal with emotionally laden subjects. Most laden, perhaps, are the process of natural death from ALS and the decisions about life-prolonging respirator and gastrostomy support; they are particularly critical in ALS because of legal uncertainties in some states about their withdrawal if the patient's condition and wishes change, and because of the implications anywhere of extending life with progressive and finally total paralysis. Many moderators feel responsible to open the subject before crisis-prompted decisions have to be made. Indeed, it is hard to find a subject related to ALS that is not emotionally charged; even the apparently all-positive subject of devices to enhance functioning is a sharp reminder of loss.

It is the processing of the emotional impact that seems to me a basis for distinguishing various support group formats: addressing the impact in varying depth, with more or less intention, with more or less personal engagement of the participants, and/or minimizing the impact through information and supportive contacts. The emphasis ranges from considerable internal coping with the disease (emotions, relationships, values, attitudes, processing information) to principally external means of coping that empower and support (information, resources, equipment, diversions, activities, projects, companionship of peers). The resulting group forms range from those closest to the group therapy model to those most distant, and any combination.

In practice, decisions about the variables that contribute to these ends are often made on a pragmatic basis: who can lead and who wants to attend. Choices that need to be made in something like this order, include:

- The membership: do you want to serve patients, caregivers or both? Together or separately? Friends and community people too?
- Do you want to present interactive discussion groups or educational programs? Programs followed by or interspersed with discussions?
- Do you intend to have ongoing continuous meetings or time-limited recurring series?
- What leadership is then appropriate and available?
- And lesser decisions that tend to fall into place.

If, however, the moderator is chosen first, most of the other decisions depend on his or her particular experience and areas of competence. The axiom is that leaders are most effective in formats with which they are professionally and personally at ease.

Leadership

In my observations, the nature of the leadership colors the nature of the group as much as any other one element. Purpose, methods, and atmosphere tend to grow out of the moderator's particular professional or lay orientation, including his or her personal philosophy and emotional grounding in relation to adversity. Stoutly-held convictions surface about what is most useful or even correct.

Mental health professionals include clinical social workers, educational counselors, psychiatrically trained nurses, and psychologists. Resources and daily management are addressed, but typically there is an added emphasis on internal coping. Method and content are adapted from therapy group models, introducing an eclectic variety of techniques to enhance functioning by resolving emotional concerns. They tend to encourage expression and resolution of "negative" feelings of guilt, anger, fear, and depression related to emotionally charged areas and to elicit recognition and resolution of maladaptive behavior and/or emotions. They may introduce subjects and techniques known to enhance relationship and communication, manage stress, or allay future regret or resentment—preventive mental health steps. I do not know of any who see the healing of overt premorbid intrapsychic disorder as appropriate to the support group, but they depend on their professional knowledge and skills to effect appropriate referral. They feel their professional knowledge and values are useful in their regard for individual differences, in eliciting concerns that are close to expression, in acceptance and openness in feeling and communication, in skill in involving or protecting group members, in encouraging member-to-member support and sharing, and in letting a group evolve according to its needs. With some luck, the leader models these values and, without interpretation, fills a reassuring transference role. Among professionals, emphasis varies depending on their position—hospice staff, sexuality counselor, medical social worker, cognitive psychologist, psychiatric nurse.

Nonpsychiatrically oriented professionals, in my observation, typically though not always emphasize external coping, drawing on mental health professionals as another valid resource among many. They see themselves supporting an action-oriented, partially (and healthily) denying style of management. Like many lay leaders, and more often than mental health professionals, they sometimes foster the members' spiritual or inspirational life as a powerful force to transcend what cannot be changed. This message may be expressed by a guest speaker, at a retreat, in reading material, or in a newsletter. They seem also more likely to encourage recreation, projects, or social get-togethers. Two groups I know of moderated by medical nurses purposely tap into a human potential that I believe may sometimes be insufficiently cultivated: an essentially robust, problem-solving, coping-oriented fortitude. Most groups have in them some patients and families, perhaps partly using the moderator as model, who accept adversity as a fact of life, expect to learn how to deal with it, and don't pay special attention to whether it meets their expectations or not. They contribute to a particular sense of normalcy and manageability.

Lay leaders express the conviction that people who have personal experience of ALS on a daily basis intuitively understand the experience in a different and truer sense than others, both the feelings and what's involved in getting through the day. Such a leader could typically be an ALS patient or caregiver or a surviving friend or relative who found no information or support available when he or she was confronting ALS. The organizer often functions as a coordinator of arrangements while the group as a whole sets agenda and direction. I have heard the view expressed, without knowing how prevalent it may be, that they feel more spontaneous without a psychologically-oriented person present who may make unwelcome (even if unexpressed) interpretations. There is an element of self-reliance, of keeping control in their own hands, with professionals of different kinds called on as they see the need. The frequent use of "ALS person" or "ALS-er," in contrast to the professional's common use of "ALS patient," seems to express this stalwart position.

My impression is that lay leaders and professionals develop cooperative and appreciative (if sometimes watchful) relationships with each other. Lay leaders have sought additional insights and skills from professionals, sometimes turning over leadership temporarily or permanently, sometimes retaining it. Most professionals I know report themselves learning as much from group members and lay leaders as they impart. They move substantially away from the medical model style of group therapy in which many were trained as specialists vis-à-vis afflicted patients and toward greater personal involvement and educational or cognitive approaches. Confronting ALS seems to bring to our attention that there is very little "we" and "they"; we all have more in common than anything that separates us, through the bond of a universal mortality and our search for fulfillment in whatever life we lead here and now.

Membership

Separate or combined groups. Another basic decision about which people entertain lively convictions is whether to have patients and caregivers in separate groups or a combined group. Lay leaders reportedly seldom consider separate groups, based on the matter-of-fact view that they're all in this together. Groups that are devoted to external means of coping are typically open to both patients and families and often community. The question arises when the format is a discussion group with some emphasis on internal means of coping or when a program is followed by discussion groups.

Supporters of separate groups point out that patients and caregivers have different issues and that separate groups permit a stronger bond of common experience and feelings. They suggest that each needs a separate place to express and explore the stressful aspects of their relationships, their "unacceptable" responses and the disappointments and demands attributable to the other. They believe that open expression is inhibited in a combined group and that these negative emotions, when unresolved or displaced, can lead to destructive behavior. (They cite in caregivers overprotection, physical illness, and harsh or negligent treatment of the patient; in patients, they cite depression, aggression, unrealistic demands, a withering of the self.) They anticipate in a combined group either avoidance of conflicting issues or irremediable hurt when issues are explored for which there is no mutually satisfactory solution in the context of ALS. On the positive side, their professional conviction is that this freer expression hastens recognition and resolution of individual emotional issues and enhances comfort, ego strengths, functioning, and relationships. It may make the problems more manageable or acceptable or open the way for freer exchange and handling of controversial subjects between the patient and the caregiver.

Among participants, caregivers more than patients seem to seek separate discussion groups; most combined groups I am aware of have in time added them in some form. My best explanation, from moderating such groups, lies in the enormous dislocation in the lives and feelings of the caregivers themselves. The buck increasingly and finally stops with them: physical care, much of the patient's former role, their own pre-ALS role, managing the changes in income and lifestyle and planning. These self-selected members used separate time (1) to take responsibility for their distinctive emotional and practical issues without adding unnecessarily to the patient's already acute sense of being a burden, (2) to address issues the patient could not or would not address with them, (3) for initial exploration of patients' moods, attitudes and behavior they did not understand (or sometimes like) or know how to respond to, (4) to anticipate and prepare themselves for hard clinical aspects of the disease, (5) to identify their own unmet needs and decide how or whether to meet them and, most importantly, (6) to learn how increasingly to communicate and address part of all of this with the patient. A principal value, I think, was to give caregivers a place to lean on others and to be nourished and refreshed.

Substantially fewer interactive patient groups were reported. They seem to be more of a challenge in a number of ways. Some patients do not want to be intimately exposed to ALS patients more advanced or differently afflicted nor to watch the progression in other patients, but numbers almost never permit a homogeneous group. Many more want information and attend the less emotionally involving groups — perhaps because more are offered. There are practical problems of accessibility, difficulty in communication, need for physical assistance for some patients, and maintaining sufficient numbers for a group. They can easily drop below five. The death of a patient is perhaps more of an assault in a group where he or she has been a well-known and active participant and where the other members can only expect the same for themselves. We should note that some leaders of patient groups report them emotionally draining because of the communication problems and because of the vivid and continual exposure to the degeneration and loss of people to whom they are professionally close.

Advocates of combined discussion groups include some mental health professionals and, notably, hospice personnel. The former see conflict resolution as their goal in groups, following a mental health model. The latter are accustomed to helping people confront the end of life together. They see it as a time when patient and family need each other, when separation should be countered, when both grieving and the development of common views and joys need to be supported: not death and dying but life and living. (A principal dynamic is the participants' willingness to regard life-expectancy as limited and therefore valuable.) It is their conviction that sharing and even confrontation open a loving, vital, and necessary way to resolution of problems. Combined-group advocates recognize that the give and take may be provocative. They counter the reservations of the separate-group advocates by screening, by referral for therapy if indicated, by occasional separate group sessions in the context of a generally shared group experience, and especially by alert and prompt individual or family intervention when unusually painful material has been unearthed. Speaking without experience in moderating a combined group, I believe it is vital that the facilitator be well-equipped to handle this kind of individual intervention as well as comfortable and skilled in handling the dynamics of confrontation in a group. The point has been made that a combined group is of unparalleled value to patients and caregivers who enjoyed a positive relationship before ALS and now seek ways to live with it together. A question occurs to me: Will the fragile functioning in a relationship that is antagonistic, distant, or at best a truce be helped or further damaged in a combined group when stresses are already exacerbated by ALS?

An occasional hybrid group combines patients in one set of families with caregivers from other families. The goal is to give each some appreciation of the other's viewpoints without addressing immediate family conflicts.

Open or closed membership. With closed membership, no new members are received after the series begins, and members commit to attend all sessions if possible. This arrangement was found only in four weekly, time-limited, recurring discussion groups, two for patients and two for caregivers, although a canvass of the many MDA groups would, I think, locate more. They had the expressed goal (along with education and daily problem-solving) of ventilation and resolution of feelings. Closed membership lends itself to confidentiality, continuity, quick coalescence, and intimate interactive relationships. It permits and calls for substantial emotional involvement. It is typical of the therapy group model.

Nearly all discussion groups allow open intermittent attendance. (They may be limited to patients or caregivers or by screening. This is selected membership but not "closed.") Moderators believe that a consistent core group develops over time with its own culture and values so that many of the goals and advantages of closed membership are retained with the added advantage of providing dependably accessible support on an as-needed basis.

For educational and resource meetings, open attendance, sometimes including interested professionals and others from the community, is almost universal, the topic often announced ahead of time so that people can self-screen.

Special populations. Inclusion in the same group of *newly-diagnosed and far-advanced patients*, or their caregivers, has emerged as a troublesome dichotomy in some discussion groups. It is clear why newcomers may be shocked and dismayed by exposure to the disease's later manifestations. A number of ways to mitigate the effect have been more or less successful: careful preparation for the group, sometimes leading to a decision to defer participation; in the more impersonal education or information-only series, provision for answering questions but not for sharing experiences; prior announcement of subject matter so people may self-screen; two or three group sessions specifically for the recently diagnosed; and stressing, within the group, the highly variable course of the disease.

What has surprised some professionals, however, is the veterans' reactions. For a while sharing with newcomers seems to reinforce the veterans' sense of themselves as capable and to give some purpose to the experiences they have endured. But at length some weary of going through it vicariously again and feel unable to address their current needs because of concern for the newcomer. Veterans have often developed close ties with group members outside the group setting and may now prefer to depend on those and individual counselling. Understandably this reaction can become a true split in the more intimate groups if the group happens to have no representatives of a middle ground with whom those at either extreme can identify—no continuum of experience. It is my impression that the philosophy of the group may also contribute to closing the gap between extremes, as when a fairly homogeneous population (unlike most large urban and suburban areas) shows a religious or cultural acceptance of adversity and death or when a hospice-sponsored group is exposed early to its very clear point of view.

Bereaved caregivers are another subgroup of concern to nearly all sponsors. Sponsors recognize that the needs of the bereaved are quite different from other group members but believe that recognition, if not ongoing support, should be offered. This may be as simple as a phone call from the moderator and individual expressions of sympathy from group members. If the moderator is prepared to do so, he or she may offer a few individual counselling sessions or referral for bereavement counselling. Often the bereaved return for one or two group sessions to share their experience of the patient's death. They bring an important set of connections to closure and confirm for themselves by their attendance that their relationship to ALS has changed, that their life will be organized around some different focus. Professionals, with their sometimes acute awareness of vulnerability, have reported their own initial uneasiness with bereaved members but have learned that this return is normally a moving and curiously reassuring experience for the group. It has seemed to me that surviving caregivers— at least those in the close-knit discussion support groups—do not require as long or as intense a working out of grief as many other survivors. Indeed this is a valuable function of a group. The survivor has often done considerable mourning in the course of ALS's continuing losses, and within the group has confronted and to some extent resolved the negative emotions ALS has stirred up. Attitudes, behavior and competencies that the survivor has cultivated during the patient's life turn out to be preparation also for self-reliant living and wholesome mourning. The bereaved may be relatively unburdened by helplessness, guilt, hostility or regrets.

Death often is seen as release for the patient and they can acknowledge it as release for themselves as well. Some survivors continue to attend; they gradually absorb their loss and find their new focus within the sponsoring multifunctional organization as lay leaders; fund raisers; visitors to the newly diagnosed, housebound, or more recently bereaved; or strong voices in increasing public awareness of ALS.

Other special populations may be accommodated separately as staffing permits. Young adult children of ALS patients or parents of young children in ALS households, for example, may attend one or two special meetings or regular meetings less frequent than those of the central group.

Method

Two general styles emerge — discussion and educational presentations — and both may be used in one program or within a series. Discussion groups lend themselves to internal means of coping. They may be planned with or without any programs, usually with occasional guest speakers as the group desires, often including a neurologist. They may have a planned agenda or topic, or follow the group's lead for the particular meeting. If the discussion group is planned to come after a program, the topic often involves processing and personalizing the program material.

Groups featuring programs usually allow for question and answer periods. They have the advantage of providing quantities of specialized information and education and they allow people as casual or as personal an involvement and as much or as little exposure to other participants' ALS experience as they wish. Unless a discussion period is provided, they carry the possibility of arousing anxiety by presenting graphic solutions to problems the patient doesn't yet have and does not want to focus on, but prior announcement allows fairly reliable self-screening. Attendance may reach 45 or 50.

Time-Limited or Open-Ended

Open-ended groups are the norm among groups sponsored by independents and ALSA. The overriding advantage is to assure ALS patients and families of a continuously available, sustaining community. The same benefit can be provided within MDA's policy of a time-limited but renewable series of meetings, if care is taken to avoid long periods between series. MDA considers the limit a useful tool to evaluate, focus, and fine-tune. In discussion groups it provides the traditional therapy advantage of encouraging participants to get their issues addressed within the designated period, lending itself especially to the weekly or biweekly forms. Some members have described the interval between series as a time to enjoy the benefits of the series and to excuse themselves for a while from focusing on the problematic aspects of their lives; others miss a continuing contact. In closed-membership groups, the time limit provides a necessary point at which new members can come in and others leave.

Publicizing and Screening

I am not aware of any sponsor who uses the general media to publicize an ALS group. The preliminary announcement is usually by letter or brochure to the roster of clinic patients or to those registered with the national office of ALSA or with the MDA local office. The newsletter of a multifunctional ALS center carries ongoing group announcements as well as general ALS news and sometimes first-person and inspirational pieces; some groups as they become established develop newsletters of their own. These have the advantage of letting people attend meetings of special interest to them and avoid those they find irrelevant or frightening. In addition, reports of meeting content reach people who cannot or prefer not to attend; they may give a sense of identification even in the absence of direct contact and they may serve as an introduction to what a support group does. Newsletters and mailings clearly entail no screening unless the instruction is to contact the moderator. Some professional facilitators feel it is desirable to reach a mutual decision with prospective attendants as to whether the group, more individualized support, therapy, or no such contact is timely for their well-being or that of the group. Some recently diagnosed patients and their families find that a sharing group provokes depression and anxiety at a time when they are managing to enjoy and use the present quite fully. Such families usually screen themselves out promptly, recognizing that the group at present does not support their adjustment. Some in full denial attend later when reality intrudes, but some are so ill-fortified for the intrusion that they rather hopelessly do not seek support. How to reach them is an unanswered question.

Frequency

The vast majority of programmed groups and many discussion groups meet monthly while some discussion groups meet weekly or twice a month. In one such group the moderators judged weekly meetings to be physically burdensome and not necessary to continuity. The more frequent meeting tends to foster continuity, intimate personal problem solving, and development of a group as distinct from an assembly of individuals. The monthly format is physically more manageable for the participants, probably less demanding emotionally, and probably provides less continuity about personal problems. It is practical if group members are widely dispersed and extensive traveling is necessary or if patients, for whom attendance involves more effort, are attending. The fee or available time of a professional moderator is also a consideration.

The most frequent time for meetings is weekday evenings, usually one and one-half to two hours. This serves family members who work days and is a time when other working family members are available to stay with the patient if needed, but it may be tiring for patients to attend at this time. Daytime meetings during the week are less frequently reported. Professional moderators are probably less available for weekend meetings, but that timing meets several needs: time to travel, time for the patient to get ready, probably the most rested time of day for the patient and time for an extended monthly program. One group, for example, meets monthly for a program at 11:00 a.m. on a Saturday, has a buffet lunch arranged by the members, and then has separate discussion groups — a day the family plans to spend together.

Meeting Places

Meeting places, as centrally located as possible and with wheelchair and bathroom accessibility for patients, include classrooms, conference rooms or cafeterias of a hospital, meeting rooms in churches and civic organizations, and homes. Patients and families have reported that comfortable, attractive surroundings added to their sense of respite and well-being.

Refreshments

Refreshments can serve a number of purposes, anything from coffee and tea with its implication of nurturing and sociability (common to most groups), through something substantial prepared by the group for an explicitly social time together, to refreshments timed after a program to encourage individual contacts. In one programmed group the refreshment hour is the opportunity for informal support among those attending and the facilitator's opportunity to see whether any individual needs or wants contact beyond the information group. In one caregivers' group the members go out for dinner to enjoy purely social time before the meeting.

FORMATS: WHAT DO THEY LOOK LIKE?

Five representative formats emerge from different combinations of these variables. Perhaps predictably, the variables tend to run in tandem as they reinforce the leadership's tilt toward internal or external resources for coping. These formats that intentionally include internal means of coping tend to be moderated by mental health professionals, use discussion method primarily, meet more often, limit size and membership and sometimes length of series, and depend on group process. Those leaning toward external reinforcement meet monthly or less often, routinely present programs, have open membership (sometimes including community people), have larger attendance, have projects and activities (often including discussion groups) that vary greatly in approach. Much administrative support – literature, announcements, letters, sometimes the meeting place, sometimes a facilitator's fee – typically comes from the local sponsoring organization.

None of these groups are seen by their members as psychotherapy groups though all are seen as therapeutic; nearly all try to provide for individual or family counseling as a necessary alternative or adjunct, by referral or within their own setting. Some people are by temperament private; some are unable and others unwilling to be exposed to different or more advanced manifestations of ALS; some suffer personality or family pathologies; others may need information and resources but consider themselves well supported by family, friends, church community. Counselors competent to address both the emotional and practical demands specific to ALS are needed for this otherwise unserved population.

Format 1

Closest to the group therapy model in form, though not following it closely in technique or content (see Leadership section), is the time-limited, weekly, closed membership, professionally-led discussion group limited to patients or caregivers and usually from 5 to 15 members in size. While it has a strong emphasis on sharing and education, it has the potential for dealing with individual emotional conflicts related to ALS, for identifying maladaptive attitudes and behavior, and for introducing alternatives from a variety of insight-oriented or behavioral theories. Its consistent membership, time limit, and frequency are seen to foster continuity; quicker coalescence into a caring cohesive group; quicker focus on concerns; freedom and safety to approach painful subjects; and maximum effectiveness of small group process. Its drawbacks are the relatively small percentage of patients and families who are prepared for this degree of commitment and emotional involvement and its lack of long-term availability to a larger ALS population. As someone who has moderated this form, I have come to believe it needs to be complemented by another consistently ongoing group in the area.

Format 2

The second, more usual format is the ongoing, monthly (or occasionally twice a month), professionally-led discussion group with open membership (though membership may be selective; i.e., limited to patients or families). Like the first format, it is self-contained, without formal agenda, projects, or activities except as the group requests a program. The group may sometimes limit a meeting to a particular population (like newcomers or adult children). In spite of fringe members and those who dip in and out, the consistent part of the membership is reported by moderators to develop into a strong, resilient, interactive group. Consequently they share method, techniques, goals, and benefits of the closed group. We do not know whether the intimacy of the closed group may be a little diluted. Until or unless such a core develops there are two possible drawbacks in my experience: (1) content may be repetitive and (2) the facilitator needs to be equipped to protect participants and the group itself from being monopolized or demoralized by the sometimes profoundly tragic outpouring of people who attend only in crisis. At that point the developing group does not have the cohesiveness to absorb and support such material. The format's pronounced advantage is its continuous accessibility as a safe haven among companions and its accommodation to whatever degree of commitment a participant wants to make.

Format 3

The third and most common format consists of ongoing monthly meetings with open membership and with a planned program most of the time, addressed to both patients and families for a substantial part of the meeting. Leadership may be by a professional explicitly or not explicitly oriented to psychotherapy (an occupational therapist, for example, often a nurse) or a nonprofessional dedicated to the cause of ALS — often a survivor, sometimes a patient. Provision is made for discussion after the program or sometimes substituting for a program. Discussants may stay in a combined group or separate into patients and caregivers, newcomers and others, with their separate lay or professional facilitators. This dependable monthly form seems to permit great flexibility in the nature of its discussion period from group to group or within the same group over time.

Depending on time allowed and the philosophy of the leadership, the discussion may focus on resources and practical problem solving with very limited continuity or focus on feelings. It may focus on processing material from the program. A discussion program on emotional and psychological aspects of ALS may be held two or three times a year, announced ahead of time to allow for self-selection. Or the discussion groups may directly deal with the more internal coping methods, although the intimacy of the discussion-only format is here somewhat attenuated, in the opinion of some leaders. One particular advantage may also be this format's possible limitation: it permits as little emotional involvement as the participant wishes and in some settings the leaders believe it does not make provision for as much involvement as some participants would like and could use. I sense, more than I can document, that some of these groups develop a particular kind of closeness; they mature into true communities with socializing and assistance among members and with members contributing to functions of the multifunctional parent organization. This sense of a broadened community in the group-plus-sponsoring-organization, its secure availability, and its flexibility in reaching different populations are substantial advantages.

Format 4

The fourth, least intense form of "support group" is the straight educational, informational program. It may be presented monthly or a few times a year, sometimes to complement the more interactive groups. It makes no effort to involve people in group process as such, but social time and attractive refreshments after the meeting are designed to encourage people to talk with each other and with the visiting or regular professionals who stay to make themselves available. One concentrated form that was presented twice, six months apart, as an "Orientation to ALS," consisted of three weekly speakers on psychosocial, medical, and legal/financial issues. There were question and answer periods each week and one follow-up meeting for those who wanted to discuss the information further. Each attracted three to four times as many as the more personally involving groups and included many people recently diagnosed or for some reason without other access to ALS peers or specialists. While a professional with group therapy background may ask if an information meeting constitutes a "group," there seems to be no question that it offers both education and supportive human contacts.

Format 5

Fifth are the self-help groups, those conducted without professional leadership. They are classed separately because lay leadership introduces a different philosophy of group participation (as discussed earlier under "Leadership") although some share many of the same practices as professionally led groups. They may arise spontaneously, sponsored by a local or national ALS organization, if a few families and patients request it after becoming acquainted at, for example, a clinic. They may be started by a clinic or other ALS community organization in an area inconvenient by distance from an existing group. While they frequently begin with guest speakers, some are reported to change to a sharing discussion group when they run out of speakers' topics and/or the members become increasingly comfortable with each other. Meetings are usually monthly, commonly with both patients and families attending. Most groups have the educational support of a larger ALS organization and may use professionals in an advisory or educational capacity, regularly or as they wish. Reservations voiced by professionals about lay-led groups (recognizing that professionals are not immune to the same issues) concern the possibilities of a strong leader consciously or unconsciously superimposing his or her own values and solutions on a group with insufficient recognition of personal differences; of highly charged emotional material leading to further anxiety and/or depression in the group rather than to resolution; and of destructive attitudes or behavior developing in or between members being either unrecognized or unaddressed by the leader. My contact with lay groups is too limited to evaluate this. They have the possibility of a much more various set of approaches and values and great potential for growth, and their variations deserve more study. The format may be as simple as a few people getting together in someone's living room or as complex as the talents, experience, and energy of particular leaders allow. Some which started very simply have developed into multifunctional centers.

SUMMARY

This is a descriptive review of representative ALS groups and choices to be made in organizing them. It is undertaken to consolidate information recently available in a supportive informal network and to encourage group planners and moderators to participate in this network. It is made up of the major group sponsors: the national offices of ALSA and MDA, their local branches, independent ALS centers and newsletters. Addresses and telephone numbers are appended.

Experience tells us that what patients and caregivers seek in a group varies: information from experts and experienced ALS people, contact with other ALS people but with differing degrees of intimacy, exploration with peers of the emotional impact and attitudes stirred by ALS.

Formats that emerge reflect this variety of needs and equally the areas of competence and comfort of available leadership. The result is some combination of two major methods—discussion or planned program. Predictably, information and daily management—the external coping resources—constitute major content in all formats.

Where groups differ in character is the degree to which they purposely address the emotional impact and attitudes—the internal coping resources—and depend on small-group dynamics. We need to make conscious choices about the variable components that shape group format and tend to contribute to a leaning toward inner or outer means of coping. Groups do not see themselves as psychotherapy for pre-ALS pathology and most offer individual and family counseling as adjunct or alternative, directly or by referral. Many offer service to special groups including bereaved caregivers.

Foremost among the variable components are the composition of the group (significantly, whether patients and caregivers meet separately or together); leadership by mental health professionals, non-psychiatrically-oriented professionals, lay leaders; discussion vis-à-vis program method; ongoing versus time-limited recurring series. Also contributing are frequency and size, screening and publicizing (including newsletters), time, place, refreshments.

Five formats are identifiable: (1) The frequent and interactive discussion groups led by mental health professionals have great potential for personal problem solving, growth, and healing. They also require the most time and emotional effort of members. With closed membership and time-limited series, they do not provide a consistently available community for the bulk of the ALS population. (2) The biweekly or monthly open membership discussion groups, usually led by mental health professionals, maintain, if they develop a core group, much of the small-group dynamics and intimacy. They provide sustained access to information and community of peers. (3) Professionally-led programs with question and answer periods combined with differing styles of discussion group and often a newsletter provide for a wide cross-section of the ALS population; less or more emotional exposure and give-and-take with peers; self-screening for announced topics; continuous access to a community; activities, projects, diversions, often involving the sponsoring organization.

(4) Regular programs every one, two, or three months, with or without question and answer periods and with planned time for informal contact with peers and professionals, are relatively simple to present, least emotionally demanding for those who attend, and appealing to many. They provide steady access to information and to contacts which participants may cultivate or not. A concentrated version of three weekly meetings has proved useful. (5) Lay-sponsored groups may use any of these formats as well as lay moderators, are often philosophically committed to self-direction, permit wide variations, and deserve their own survey. Professionals and laypeople are benefiting from each other's accumulated experience.

CONCLUSION

The review confirms that each format attracts its own population. This natural fit means that all groups are valid and will serve some part of the ALS population well. We need to understand that there may be an unserved population ready for a complementary style of group to be presented as our resources allow. I have come to believe that the essential element is assurance of consistent sustaining access to a community of peers and professionals while ALS patients and families seek out competence, confidence and control and a new kind of hope to put ALS in its place within a valued life.

REFERENCE

Powell, T. J. 1986. *Self-Help Organizations and Professional Practice*. National Association of Social Workers, 7981 Eastern Ave., Silver Springs, MD 20910.

ADDITIONAL READING

Finger, S. 1987. "The Family Support Group in the Treatment of Amyotrophic Lateral Sclerosis." *Neurologic Clinics* 5(1).

Kitto, J. R. and K. Garry. 1984. "A Model for Information and Support to the Amyotrophic Lateral Sclerosis Patient." *Archives of the Foundation of Thanatology* 11(2).

Leach, C. F. and J. Kelemen. 1987. "The Role of Family Groups in the Support Network for Amyotrophic Lateral Sclerosis." In Leon I. Charash et al., eds., *Realities in Coping with Progressive Neuromuscular Diseases*. Philadelphia: Charles Press.

RESOURCES

Readings

Finger, Sandra: "The Family Support Group in the Treatment of Amyotrophic Lateral Sclerosis," *Neurologic Clinics*, Vol. 5, No. 1, February 1987.

Update through author:	and Muscular Dystrophy Association:
Sandra Finger, MSW	MDA
33 River Road	450 Washington Street
RFD South Deerfield, MA 01373	Dedham, MA 02026
	Marcia Randall
	Patient Service Coordinator

Group Form II, MDA Affiliation

Kitto, J. R. and Garry, K.: "A Model for Information and Support to the Amyotrophic Lateral Sclerosis Patient," *Archives of the Foundation of Thanatology*, Vol. 11, No. 2, 1984, (The Foundation of Thanatology, 630 West 168th Street, New York, NY 10032).

Update through Muscular Dystrophy Association
4530 West 77th Street, Suite 164
Minneapolis, MN 55435
(612) 832-5517
Carol Hennon, Personal Service Coordinator

Group Form III, MDA Affiliation

Leach, C. F. and Kelemen, J.: "The Role of Family Groups in the Support Network for Amyotrophic Lateral Sclerosis," *Realities in Coping with Progressive Neuromuscular Diseases*, Leon I. Charash et al., Editors, (The Charles Press Publishers, Inc., 1987—P.O. Box 15715, Philadelphia, PA, 19103).

Update through author:
Claire F. Leach, MSW
Department of Neurology
Nassau County Medical Center
East Meadow, NY 11554
(516) 542-3107

Group Forms I (separate caregiver group) and IV, MDA Affiliation

Powell, Thomas J., *Self-Help Organizations and Professional Practice*, National Association of Social Workers, 1986.

Available through NASW
7981 Eastern Avenue
Silver Springs, MD 20910
Attention Publication Sales

Toll Free Number 1-800-638-8799

National Organizations

The ALS Association
21021 Ventura Boulevard, #321
Woodland Hills, CA 91364
(818) 340-7500
Lynn M. Klein
Director of Patient Services
Publication: *Link*

Muscular Dystrophy Association
810 Seventh Avenue
New York, NY 10019
(212) 586-0808
Ronald J. Schenkenberger
Director of Patient and Community Services
Publication: *Eye on ALS*

National Self-Help Clearinghouse
Graduate School and University Center of the City
University of New York
33 West 42nd Street, Room 620N
New York, NY 10036
(212) 642-2944
Dr. Frank Riefsman, Director
Publications: *How to Start a Self-Help Group*, booklet
              Self-Help Reporter, periodical

Sponsoring Organizations

ALS Health Support Services
(Independent)
12815 N.E. 124th, Suite "I"
Kirkland, WA 98034
(206) 821-7955   GROUP FORMS II
ALS HSS Newsletter   AND V

ALS & Neuromuscular Research Foundation
(Independent)
2351 Clay Street, Suite 416
San Francisco, CA 94115
(415) 923-3604
Newsletter   GROUP FORM III

Les Turner ALS Foundation, Ltd.
(Independent)
3325 West Main Street
Skokie, IL 60076   GROUP FORM II
(312) 679-3311   (Separate patient &
Happenings   family groups)

ALS of Michigan, Inc.
(Independent)
19111 West 10 Mile Road, Suite 203
Southfield, MI 48075   GROUP FORMS I
(313) 352-3070   (Separate patient
Reaching Out   group) and III or IV

Keith Worthington ALS Society
(Independent; became ALSA Chapter,
Spring, 1988)
8340 Mission Road, Suite B-10
Shawnee Mission, KS 66206
(913) 648-2062   GROUP FORM III
Dialog   WITH VARIATIONS

Cleveland Clinic Support Group
ALSA Eastern Ohio Chapter
c/o Mrs. Sally Nousek
4971 Countryside Road   GROUP FORMS III
Lyndhurst, OH 44124   OR IV
Letter   (Lay Sponsorship)

ALSA Upstate NY Support Group
315 South Manning Boulevard
Albany, NY 12208   GROUP FORMS II
(518) 454-1629   AND III
ALS Newsletter   (Hospice Affiliation)

ALSA Greater Philadelphia Chapter
P.O. Box 507   GROUPS II, III
Norristown, PA 19404   AND V
(215) 277-3508   (Some combined
ALS News   discussion groups)

ALSA Southern Florida Chapter
P.O. Box 4651
Margate, FL 33063   GROUP FORM II
(305) 971-6427   OR IV
ALS Talks   (Lay leadership)

ALSA Greater St. Louis Chapter
3945 West Pine Boulevard
St. Louis, Missouri 63108
(314) 534-0610   GROUP FORM III
ALS News and Views   OR IV

ALSA Orange County Chapter
13772 Goldenwest, #237
Westminster, CA 92683
(714) 962-7928   GROUP FORM II
Reaching Out   OR III

ALSA Western Pennsylvania Chapter
P.O. Box 2127
Pittsburgh, PA 15230-2127   GROUP FORM III
(412) 521-5759   OR IV
ALS News & Views   (Lay Sponsorship)

Muscular Dystrophy Association
4800 S.W. Macadam Avenue
Suite 112
Portland, OR 97201
Patricia Helzer,
Patient Service Coordinator   GROUP FORM IV

ALS Support Group of Rhode Island
Hospice Care of Rhode Island   GROUP FORMS II
345 Blackstone Boulevard   AND III
Providence, RI 02906   (Combined Group,
(401) 272-4900   Hospice Affiliation)

Comprehensive Care
for ALS Patients and Families

Bonnie Sutter
Edward Dick

At St. Peter's Hospice, we recognize the need for an individualized, comprehensive plan to address the needs of amyotrophic lateral sclerosis (ALS) patients and their families. The first ALS patient was seen in 1982; since that time, the hospice has served 45 ALS patients and their families. Most of these referrals have come to us in the last three years. The MDS refers 64 percent of these patients, 29 percent are referred by physicians, and other agencies account for the remaining eight percent. In May of 1986, a patient and family support group was started, and in July of 1987, this group became part of the National ALS Association's network of support groups. We are currently following 20 patients with the diagnosis of ALS, 13 of whom participate in the support group along with friends or family members. Seven patients participate in the day care program, and one is currently on the home care service.

A team approach is essential in providing a supportive system to foster a sense of hopefulness in patients and their families, while dealing with the deteriorating progression of the disease. Not only the physical needs of the patient must be addressed, but also the psychological and spiritual needs. The hospice team is available to ALS patients and their families to provide a wide range of services, including nursing care, pastoral care, bereavement coordination, social work, occupational therapy, and volunteer services, as well as psychiatry. Group and individual situations are utilized to provide support and share information.

While hospice staff have provided ALS patients with supportive care during the end stage of their illness, the ALS support group serves a wide range of ALS patients of varying levels of disability. The need for addi-

Bonnie Sutter, OTR, is Hospice Day Care Coordinator, and Edward Dick, ACSW, is Psychospiritual Coordinator at St. Peter's Hospice, Albany, NY 12203.

tional services has been identified to provide comprehensive care to the ALS patient from diagnosis through the end stages of the disease. While MDS clinics, rehabilitation departments, hospices, and other health care programs and personnel provide valuable services to ALS patients and families, they are not designed to provide a comprehensive system of support from diagnosis to death.

We are currently developing a regional ALS center that will make available to the patient a most comprehensive system of support throughout the course of the disease. Early referrals will be encouraged. The initial evaluation would be made by the interdisciplinary team. Members will include a nurse, a physical therapist, an occupational therapist, a speech therapist, and a social worker. We will evaluate the need for volunteers. Following a team meeting, a written plan of care will be developed. Follow-up will include the following:

Home visit. For those patients living within a one-hour driving distance, a home visit can provide the health care professional the opportunity to view patients in their home environment, recommend home modifications or assistive devices, and instruct patients in a home exercise program. The home visit also provides a conducive setting for family teaching.

Inpatient admission. An inpatient admission to the rehabilitation unit may be indicated during the early stage of the disease to initiate a therapy program. During a short-term admission, the patient can be instructed in an exercise program to maintain the integrity of unaffected musculature while learning compensation and energy conservation techniques to accommodate for lost function. Adapted equipment to compensate for functional losses could also be provided.

Outpatient services. Outpatient services may include speech therapy, physical therapy, and respiratory therapy. The clinic is also available to the outpatient where such services as pulmonary testing may be needed.

Home care follow-up. Follow-up care, as appropriate, may be offered via St. Peter's Home Care, St. Peter's Hospice, or a referral to a home care or hospice in the patient's community.

ALS Clinic. Regularly scheduled clinic visits and participation in the support group also provide follow-up.

Day care. The day care program also allows for continued contact as well as providing the patient with respite care, training in activities of daily living (ADL), socialization, and the opportunity to participate in a prayer group or activity group. A whirlpool is available for pain control or hygiene. Training in relaxation techniques and massage are also available for pain control or to decrease anxiety. The day care program is located in St. Peter's Hospital, therefore related services are readily available.

ALS support group. The ALS support group meets once monthly for one and one-half hours, for the purpose of education as well as support to the patient and family. Topics include exercise, dietary needs, relaxation training, discussion of life support systems, family coping, and question and answer sessions. A typical group may include five to ten patients, with or without their families. Also in attendance are family members who live out of town, hospice and hospital staff who work with ALS patients, and occasional health care workers from outlying areas who are working with ALS patients. Sessions are videotaped and loaned out to patients who miss a session. Most patients are receptive to participating in the videotaping, as they become the teachers in this situation and achieve a renewed sense of self-esteem through this role. A camaraderie forms among the members who are eager to share and learn from each other. A sense of comfort and support is derived from being in the company of others who can understand the vicissitudes of coping with ALS on a day-to-day basis. Fears and concerns can be openly expressed.

ALS clinic. A follow-up visit at the ALS clinic occurs at regular intervals, involving both the patient and family. A reevaluation is completed at this time, and problem areas are addressed.

Phone contact. Patients are encouraged to contact staff via telephone with any problems or questions. In addition, volunteer and paid staff maintain regular contact with patients. Volunteer contact can be an integral part of the care plan.

Our background in hospice work provides us with good experience in dealing with the patient who expresses a progressive deterioration of functional abilities. A well-organized plan of care designed by the ALS team can provide the patient and family with necessary medical management as well as the psychological support needed to continue as purposeful and meaningful a lifestyle as possible.

A core concept in the formulation of this comprehensive care center for the ALS patient is the provision of ongoing psychosocial and spiritual care. What distinguishes this concept from other comprehensive care constructs is the notion that all of the interdisciplinary team members as well as the patient/family unit are seen as potential psychosocial and spiritual caregivers.

Part of what makes ALS such a difficult disease is the relentless suffering of loss upon loss without benefit of the traditional hope systems — the hope for cure, the hope chemotherapy provides the cancer patient for prolongation of his life, the hope of a heart patient that surgery might cure his illness. There is no treatment shown to stop, slow, or modify ALS disease progress.

Thus the need for a transformation of what is "hopeful" for the patient and family becomes vital from the time of diagnosis and remains paramount through the course of the disease.

The ALS patient and family need multiple and varied opportunities to talk about what the illness means to them. It becomes the task of the entire team to be open to these opportunities when they arise. The clinic environment becomes, in essence, a milieu in which a patient, finding he or she wants to talk during a whirlpool, will be encouraged to do so; or the cues of a family member over coffee that he or she is feeling overwhelmed will be responded to by whatever team member is with her. These informal opportunities, coupled with more traditional counseling, prove crucial in helping the patient/family unit maintain some sense of mastery and control over their lives. With a sense of mastery and control comes a condition that I call hopefulness.

When the ALS patient and family are given opportunities to find meaning in the illness, and can take advantage of these opportunities, besides a renewed sense of mastery and hopefulness comes another benefit. The patient and family can now be more clear about the decisions they need to make. Very important decisions about experimental treatment, life support systems, G-tubes, rehabilitation, etc., are freed from the sense of desperation that may otherwise accompany them. There is a context now in which to make decisions.

When this process is not engaged with the ALS patient and family, few are able to establish it themselves. Many patients and families wander about in a quandary, searching desperately for cures, collecting bits and pieces of information and misinformation, feeling isolated and alone, and operating from an often shaky set of premises about both the disease and themselves. Even when there are multiple systems involved with the patient and family, the lack of an overall philosophy and closely coordinated effort may contribute to the sense of fragmentation the patient and family feel. The opportunity for the ALS patient and family to talk about the illness, to search for meaning and a sense of mastery and control over their lives is essential for the ability to make good and appropriate choices about their treatment and their living.

One of the important ways in which St. Peter's Hospice has attempted to help patients and families find meaning is the ALS support group. Facilitated by the hospice day care coordinator and the hospice social worker, the goal of the support group is multifaceted. Support and education are the primary functions. But what is extremely important is the recognition and utilization of patients and families as knowledgeable resources. A conscious attempt is made to soften reliance on medical systems for all the answers and directions. Using Swartz's Mutual Aid Model (Shulman 1980), the facilitators take advantage of opportunities to get patients and families talking with, sharing ideas with, and supporting each other. While our support group topics are valuable in providing the context of specifically needed information on nutrition, exercise, relaxation, disease etiology, etc., it is the discussion that takes place among us as a group, among patients and families in particular, that lies at the heart of the group's benefit. ALS patients and families are an incredible resource for each other.

On one level is the sharing of information regarding day-to-day management, assistive devices, foods, adaptive clothing, what works, what doesn't work. There is a wealth of information shared.

On another level is the sharing of frustration, of hope, of humor, and of tears. At our most recent ALS support group meeting, a patient named Ed was discussing his reluctance to travel to Florida this winter as he had done in past years. Ed is currently quite independent—able to care for himself, drive, and engage in a variety of home management activities. Another patient in the group, Pedro, was lying on a couch as he is without use of either hands or legs and cannot sit up on his own. He told Ed of his intention to revisit his homeland of Puerto Rico in the next month. Another patient, Andy, wheelchair-bound, unable to clearly speak or use his hands, managed to communicate to Ed his intentions to go to Florida this winter with his wife. Bolstered by these stories, Ed changed his mind and decided to make the trip. If these more disabled men could meet their challenges, then he could meet his.

Another more stirring story of hope and perseverance came from a woman, Mary Eleanor, who, wheelchair-bound and with 50 percent loss of hand function, woke up one night in her home unable to sleep, so she got herself out of bed, into her wheelchair, and out to her adapted kitchen. There she spent the next six hours laboriously making two lemon meringue pies for her family. Her story was told with joy. There was humor at the mess she made, pride in her perseverance, and hopefulness that lay in being present to the moment in these six hours, living them as fully as she had ever lived.

These stories are the heart of what makes the support groups beneficial for all involved. Through stories such as these and through the interaction of the ALS patients and families in the group lies the search for personal meaning.

With the social worker's background in group work and nearly 12 years of combined experience by the facilitators viewing patients and families as the unit of care in hospice work, it seemed fitting and natural to include patients and families together in the ALS support group. Whether consciously or unconsciously, an ALS diagnosis brings with it the threat of death and a fear of loss of physical and emotional control. Protecting ourselves and our families from these worries and fears works to keep us stuck, unable to integrate what the disease means. It also isolates us from our closest support system — each other.

By including both patients and families in group discussion we send the message that it is not only all right but important that they learn about the illness and share it together. Furthermore, in a group, patients and families can model for each other new ways of being open with their families and coping with the disease. We cannot take away another's suffering. We can only bear witness that the suffering is real and be available to each other. In the family lies the greatest source of support and coping. By including and mobilizing this resource, by giving the family some direction, education, and emotional and spiritual support, we most fully service the ALS patient.

REFERENCE

Shulman, L. 1980. *The Skills of Helping Individuals and Groups*. Springfield, IL: F. E. Peacock Publishers.

ADDITIONAL READING

Bowlby, J. 1973. *Attachment and Loss, Vol. II: Separation*. New York: Basic Books.
Feifell, H., ed. 1977. *New Meanings of Death*. New York: McGraw-Hill.

China's Care of the Disabled

Dennis Ryan

China just recently completed its first census of the disabled in over 40 years. The survey projects that there are 51.6 million disabled persons. The results are based on interviews with more than one and a half million people in 424 countries and cities throughout China. The World Health Organization provided support for the project. The study intends to identify various groups of handicapped people, as well as the causes of their disabilities; their family, employment, and social situation; and their medical care. Prior to the release of the findings, China estimated that the number of the handicapped was only about 20 million (Beijing Review, 1987).

But what is the care that is available to these people now? Are they left on their own? Is this lack of knowledge of their numbers indicative of the government's lack of care?

China does not like foreigners to learn of its shortcomings. Information, especially if it might be construed as damaging to China's world image, is difficult to obtain. However, living in China for a year might yield some clues to these questions and others. For the academic year, from September 1985 to August 1986, I lived in Dalian, in Liaoning Province in the Northeast of China. I taught students majoring in foreign trade at the Northeast University of Finance and Economics. This essay is based primarily on first-hand observation and personal interviews I conducted during the period. Therefore, my study is neither comprehensive nor representative of all of China. My observations and interviews were, for the most part, limited to the area where I lived and worked. Nevertheless, I present what I think is an informative glimpse into this aspect of health care in China today.

When foreigners with handicaps travel in China, they are alarmed by the absence of means to make their journey less arduous. Ramps as alter-

Dennis Ryan, PhD, is Associate Professor of Religious Studies, College of New Rochelle, New Rochelle, NY 10805.

233

natives to steps and stairs are nonexistent; elevators are very few. Doors, instead of yielding easily to the push of a child or elderly person, require Herculean effort, making them impossible for the handicapped. These and other helps for the handicapped just are not in place. In fact, a delegation of handicapped people from the United States visited China in 1986 and criticized the woeful lack of access to public transportation for all the handicapped, not just visitors (*New York Times* September 7, 1986).

If the government is not helping, whom are they to turn to for aid? The handicapped and infirm, in China, primarily rely on family. Family support has been a characteristic of Chinese society and culture for thousands of years, going back to the teachings of Confucius. Taking care of family members who cannot take care of themselves is the source of traditional social status and esteem. This is not only true of grown children caring for their aged parents, but also parents taking care of growing children who have handicaps or disabilities.

One of my students spoke highly of his parents in this regard. Her brother was born when she was four years old. As the child grew, the parents noticed that he walked abnormally and took him to the local "doctor," who was more like a paramedic. He suggested that the parents take their son to the nearest big city, to a hospital, and have the child examined by those doctors. My student's family is part of the 75-80 percent of China's one billion plus population that lives in the countryside. The doctors in the city hospital told the parents there was nothing they could do for the boy. So the parents took him back home and cared for him until he died at about the age of 16. He had become progressively weaker and when he could no longer walk, they would have to carry him about. My student didn't know what the disease her brother had was called, however she remembered that, as death approached, he had trouble breathing. Her brother had never gone to school, but she had managed to teach him the basics of reading and writing Chinese.

All my students reflected certain Chinese attitudes toward health and sickness. First, health is a responsibility and each person should take responsibility for his or her health. Second, when someone gets sick, it is nature that will cure the person, so the task of the caregivers is to care for them gently, in the best possible atmosphere to promote healing. And, finally, if the patient does not recover his or her health, that is fate and should be accepted. These attitudes were almost unanimously confirmed by my students.

Near the school where I taught was a medical college and hospital, and there were over 700 medical students there. There was also an American woman teaching these students English. This woman, Marcia, was my access to this institution, its practices, and the attitudes of the young medical students.

The medical students were taught about diseases such as muscular dystrophy and used the most up-to-date textbooks in English. What they were able to do with the information was greatly limited by their very limited resources. In one of her classes, Marcia posed my student's brother as a hypothetical case to be discussed as an oral English exercise. She learned that there would be no braces given, nor surgery offered, nor even physiotherapy to correct contractures and to preserve mobility. Nor would there be any genetic counseling. If this were an only child, then the couple would qualify to have another child. The reason for this exception to the one-child law is that the child with the disease would not be able to support his parents in their old age. When Marcia pressed them whether they would inform the parents of the risk that the next child might also carry the disease, her students were reluctant to put this anxiety in the mind of the couple. They would face that sorrow when, and if, it came. Amniocentesis would be prohibitively expensive; telling them would only give them worries.

There were some treatments the medical students said they would recommend, but these were drawn from traditional Chinese medicine. For example, they said they would recommend acupressure massage. Massage units are not only part of the treatment of some disabilities but the services are often rendered by the blind, and some claim to have curative, not just palliative, powers. They would also recommend some traditional exercises to keep Qi, the vital energy, flowing through the patient's body. And finally, they would recommend some foods and traditional drugs to keep them from getting constipated.

The lack of orthopedic appliances for handicapped people was disturbing, but true. I never saw any wheelchairs outside the hospital, nor, for that matter, any ambulances. People were brought to the hospital either on the bus or a bicycle or some other vehicle such as a wheelbarrow. I did observe a few hand-powered adult tricycles for the handicapped. When I asked how these were made available, I was told that families that could afford it would contract with a metal worker to make such a vehicle. When I inquired about these at local bike shops, I was told that they did not sell them but that individuals could have them specially made. During my year in China, I saw only about six such vehicles.

The Chinese government admits that it cannot afford the expense of caring for its disabled. Therefore, it encourages work units to form welfare enterprises, to offer employment and social opportunities for them. There are an estimated 28,000 of these, mostly in larger cities. It is reported that during the sixth Five-Year Plan period, various organizations under the Ministry of Civil Affairs provided jobs for 344,889 disabled.

In Dalian, there were enterprises where the disabled were employed. These varied in size, employing as few as a dozen and as many as 208. These businesses were run either by a voluntary neighborhood committee, whose members were drawn from the retired older citizens living in the area, or by large factories or other work units. Often, if a work unit was big enough, there would be enough children and relatives of the workers who were disabled to motivate such an enterprise. The Dalian Railway Workers Unit is a good example. They organized a services company to provide jobs for 80 percent of the 260 disabled children of its employees. These services included cleaning, sewing, and laundry services. A wool sweater company was also set up.

Another much smaller enterprise was started by a neighborhood committee for a combination of elderly and handicapped residents. Together, under the management of some retired workers, they made souvenirs from sea shells to be sold to the many tourists, mostly Chinese, who come to this seaside city to escape the inland heat of summer. Profits made from the enterprise helped supplement state food allowances for the handicapped. A day care center for handicapped children was also organized by another neighborhood committee. Modest fees were charged to help supplement the pensions of the retired workers who ran the facility. They even organized a match-making service to help handicapped people meet socially.

The recent census of the handicapped, identifying these people and their needs, was the latest step by the government to help these people. China knows that there is much more that is needed in the way of medical and social services. But these services are taking a back seat to efforts to modernize the economy of China. The modernizations do include upgrading China's aging technical medical equipment and improving the scientific learning of its health care personnel, but something like services for the handicapped is not a priority. It is not true that the government does not care. It does, but its priorities now are to improve the economy so that eventually, through tax revenues and foreign income, it will be able to do more for the nation's disabled. Until then, it encourages grass roots efforts like those described above.

In conclusion, as the United States faces its responsibility for the huge budget deficit it has accumulated, it will have to make decisions about priorities similar to those China has had to make. If cuts in health and social services to reduce spending are inevitable, then we will need to look to the private sector even more to help those who have special needs. China's efforts seem strikingly like some advocated in our society. For example, we need to use the wisdom, experience, and skills of our retired elderly. More value should be placed on more realistic treatment of symptoms than on expensive research, which we can no longer afford. In looking for possible compromises, we would do well to look at China and how she is handling the services for over a billion people with resources that are only a fraction of our own.

REFERENCES

Beijing Review. December 21, 1987, pp. 11-12.
Beijing Review. January 26, 1987, pp. 19-23.
New York Times. September 7, 1986.

Hoping Strategies for the Amyotrophic Lateral Sclerosis Patient

Tae-Sook Kim

INTRODUCTION

Amyotrophic lateral sclerosis (ALS) is a rapidly progressing disease of the central nervous system affecting anterior horn cells of the spinal cord. The average prognosis, after diagnosis, is two to five years. Patients suffer many symptoms during the process of the illness such as muscle weakness, fatigue, fasciculations, cramps, and spasticity, in addition to difficulties in swallowing, speaking and breathing.

After the diagnosis of ALS was established, it was found that patients' primary concerns were of an existential nature. Concerns for the future, and concerns about death, were often expressed by many patients. Individuals afflicted with ALS are reminded acutely of their unavoidable mortality each time they experience further physical deterioration. Many individuals with ALS are tempted by despair and, as a result, often adopt a defeatist or passive attitude early in treatment or as treatment progresses. Experiences of functional losses, disturbing physical symptoms, relentless progression, in addition to painful awareness of the physical deterioration, knowing that there is no proven cure for ALS and it will only get worse, are more than enough factors to contribute to the individual feeling overwhelmed and hopeless.

Tae-Sook Kim, RN, MSN, CNRN, is Research Nurse Clinician, Department of Education Research and Development, Amyotrophic Lateral Sclerosis Research Center, Columbia Presbyterian Medical Center, 710 West 168th Street, New York, NY 10031.

The author wishes to thank the MDA of New York City for its support of the Eleanor and Lou Gehrig MDA/ALS Support Group at the Columbia Presbyterian Medical Center. Special thanks to Pregrine Murphy for editorial assistance on this paper.

This paper will explore the role of hope in living with ALS and will consider a few practical methods that can be utilized by caregivers in order to assist ALS patients in restoring and maintaining hope in their daily lives.

The concept of hope is defined many ways. The ancient Greeks used the term hope in reference to a somewhat ambiguous and open-ended future. The Chinese word for hope symbolizes something rare but very precious, which is found in the future. In religious terms, hope refers to a positive expectation and fervent desire. Silvia Lange (1978) defines hope as a collection of feelings and thoughts centering on the belief that there are solutions to needs and problems.

While hope as a concept is rather difficult to define, there is general agreement that having hope leads one to feel positive, confident, secure, optimistic, comforting, encouraged, and reassured. When one has hope, one feels that life is worth living in spite of all its troubles. Each person's idea of hope is highly individual however, and assures unique meaning for the individual, but at the same time, it is a commonly shared human experience. While hope is directed to the future, it is possible to experience hope in one's life here on earth. Hope is one of the most powerful resources of a human being. An individual's level of hope determines whether human beings live or die.

There are various methods that can be utilized in order to promote hope in ALS patients. Wright's framework is presented as a paradigm of an individual's system of hope. Wright (1968) describes four cognitive-affective tasks that are present in the hoping process. These four tasks include reality surveillance, encouragement, worrying and mourning. The first task is cognitive; the other three are affective. The cognitive component of hope reflects the individual's idea of hope in conjunction with their perceived perception of reality. The affective component of hope refers to emotions arising from the individual as a result of the feelings of equilibrium or balance obtained from the cognitive component of hope. The methods that can be utilized, in order to promote hope in ALS patients, fall within the cognitive component of hope. Those methods encompass such aspects as: environmental conditions, inventory of patient's assets and abilities, growth possibilities (growing edges), group comparison, consensual validation, personal responsibility, negative avoidance, conditional events, speculative coercion of reality, future possibilities, truism, hope commendation, testimonial, and unpromising future. A description of these aspects follows:

1. ENVIRONMENTAL CONDITIONS

Environmental conditions are found to support a realistic basis of hope. These conditions of hope can either be in the present or in the future. Since an individual's immediate environment varies, it is suggested that environmental conditions that are applicable to all ALS patients should be examined. For an illness like ALS, patients and family need external help and support. While it is true that the cure for ALS has not been found, there are different medical therapies and supportive managements available. Since features of ALS vary highly among patients, management of individual ALS cannot be generalized.

The subtle nature of symptom development and the variety of disease manifestations sometimes make the diagnosis of ALS extremely difficult. In fact, there are people who are misdiagnosed at the onset and subsequently remain untreated until treatment modalities are no longer effective. For example, the symptoms of ALS (motor neuron disease) and multifocal motor neuropathy are quite similar and must be diagnosed very carefully. Neuromuscular specialists are medical experts who treat patients afflicted with ALS. However, neuromuscular specialists are often difficult to locate and can be quite costly. Therefore, individuals are sometimes hesitant to consult these specialists.

One example of an extremely effective external support agency is the Muscular Dystrophy Association (MDA). While ALS is a motor neuron disease and not a muscular dystrophy, MDA does support the care, treatment and research of ALS. MDA is one of the nation's largest voluntary health agencies and provides comprehensive services to ALS patients. Some of the ways in which MDA promotes external support and care to ALS patients and their families include: Initial diagnostic services; therapeutic services; and rehabilitation follow-up. These services are offered by neuromuscular disease specialists at the MDA-supported ALS clinics. It is important to note that if one does not have private or public insurance, the cost of the visit to the MDA-supported ALS clinic is covered by the MDA. With respect to rehabilitative follow up, MDA assists in the payment of physical therapy, for up to twelve sessions annually when prescribed by a clinic physician, and assists in the payment of up to four visits annually for occupational therapy, which aids individuals in maximum use of their remaining physical capabilities, by learning to utilize specially-designed equipment. MDA provides assistance with respiratory therapy, which may be prescribed to either augment or increase vital lung capacity. Another important way in which MDA helps ALS patients is with the purchase, rental or repair of orthopedic equipment, when prescribed by the clinic physician. These items include walkers, selected braces, wheelchairs, hospital beds, suction machines, bathing aids, and hydraulic lifts. Similarly, MDA assists with the purchase, rental and repair of aids to enhance independence in daily living, including, items like long-handle reachers, book holders, writing aids, and zipper pulls.

These medical services are furnished to ALS patients through MDA's patient service program. There are approximately 240 MDA clinics nationwide. Locations of these local MDA clinics can be obtained by calling the MDA's local chapters or by contacting the national office at 342 Madison Avenue, New York, NY 10173 or at (212) 557-8450. As was mentioned earlier, in addition to providing medical care and support services to ALS patients, MDA also contributes significantly to research for ALS. MDA research investigates promising leads in hopes of a cure for ALS, and funds promising experimental treatments, that might slow, stop or reverse the progression of the disease.

2. INVENTORY OF THE ASSETS AND ABILITIES ATTRIBUTED TO ALS

As ALS progresses in an individual, attributes vary from patient to patient. Assisting or monitoring the patient with a realistic assessment of their attributes can also serve to promote and maintain hope. Encouraging the patient to ask such questions as, "What are my good points?" or "What is special about me?" will help one to focus in this aspect. Individuals with ALS will often realize that they have many positive attributes after an interview such as this. What exactly are the attributes associated with ALS? First, some positive physical aspects of ALS. While weakness in ALS involves all skeletal muscles (voluntary muscles), it also spares several functions. The muscles controlling the eyes are often not affected, or at the very least, are not affected until very late in the disease process. Consequently, when the muscles involving the throat are affected, which then inhibits speech, the movement of the eyes makes communication possible, even when there are no other muscle movements available to the patient. Voluntary control of the sphincters of bladder and rectum enables the patient to control urine and bowel movements. Sexual functions are also not affected. The sensory functions such as seeing, hearing, smelling, tasting and feeling are not affected, as well as the intellectual capacity. Therefore, even though individuals may be diagnosed with ALS, they can still think, feel, love, communicate, maintain bladder and bowel continence and enjoy sex. Additionally, if the patients are physically healthy before their diagnosis of ALS, they probably will be in an even better position to assess their attributes realistically, and maintain their physical attributes longer. Interpersonal attributes involve the ALS patient's personal relationships with family, friends and other people in the community and can be pursued in how the patient identifies and clarifies his/her role function within that community. In terms of role function potentials, each person continues with his/her role as a member of society. Being diagnosed with ALS does not change one's status as a family member or as a person. One is still a father, mother, wife, husband, sister, brother, son or daughter. It is important to note that the ALS patient is not a disabled person, but a person who happens to be disabled. One can still fulfill individual roles successfully in spite of having ALS, by actively participating in interpersonal, family, or community discussions and by maintaining one's responsibility in decision making.

3. GROWTH FORCES

Progression in disease development can offer the ALS patient opportunities to explore various growing edges. Patients learn how to take their time in doing tasks because of the loss of muscle coordination. Additionally, ALS patients learn how to manage time and conserve energy in order to respond to the fatigue that is prompted by ALS. Patients also discover how to refine focusing and concentration, as even the simplest activity, such as swallowing or walking, requires total concentration. Consequently, they learn how not to do two things at the same time, such as talking and swallowing, or talking and walking. These learning opportunities often stimulate the ALS patient to discover and claim hidden gifts and abilities that might otherwise have remained unclaimed. These newly explored areas enable the ALS patient to view the unexplored areas of life as an opportunity for personal growth and possible happiness.

4. GROUP COMPARISON

The attributes of an individual with ALS can be verified through group demonstration and comparison. ALS patients oftentimes demonstrate a need to compare the progression of their disease, coping mechanisms, external support, and medical management with other ALS patients. Quite often patients are relieved to discover that they are coping as well, or even better, than other people with the same condition. Opportunities for group comparison can be found at ALS clinics and ALS support groups. `

5. CONSENSUAL VALIDATION OF FEELINGS

The emotions that are manifested in ALS patients are often frustration, anger, fear, depression and grief. These feelings need to be recognized. Recognition of these feelings by people around the patient, family members, friends and caregivers, often follow subtle, and sometimes not so subtle, signs or manifestations of the patient's attitude or behavior. It is important that discussion of these feelings be encouraged and acknowledged by the patient's family, friend, and care givers. Statements such as, "You look depressed today" or "Why are you not using your Ankle Foot Orthosis (AFO) for your right foot when you walk?" will help the person to bring his feelings or activities into focus and open up discussion. In these discussions, the most important consideration is in establishing and maintaining a clear communication channel. If however, the patient does not have a supportive interpersonal environment encompassed by friends or family who assist the patient in discussing feelings and behaviors, the ALS patient can still participate in this activity through self-reflection. Simply looking into a mirror and evaluating one's appearance on a regular basis may be one way to recognize, and acknowledge these feelings.

Consensual validation, therefore, can be one method in establishing communication between the patient and the supportive interpersonal environment. Consensual validation can also assist with preventative intervention. Some ALS patients have great difficulty in accepting help from assistive devices, such as wheelchairs, and consequently resist rehabilitative treatment. Oftentimes, unrealistic fears that remain unverbalized contribute significantly to the resistance of rehabilitative treatment. Encouraging communication regarding rehabilitation and supportive care can help in reducing resistance and many detrimental falls, causing additional injuries, can be prevented when ALS patients accept appropriate assistance when needed.

6. PERSONAL RESPONSIBILITY

There is a positive correlation between a degree of hope and a positive perception of reality. Favorable reality perception can be promoted by ALS patients assuming greater responsibility for their personal care. Additionally, an internal sense of control can also be maintained, in most situations, if the patient assumes greater responsibility in personal care. Family members and health care providers can only care for the patient. The effect of that care is heavily influenced by the reception of the patient. Thus, the ultimate responsibility for positive medical management lies with the ALS patients themselves. Therefore, it is very important that the ALS patient assume as much responsibility as possible in medical decision making and management.

7. AVOIDING NEGATIVE POSSIBILITIES

Hope is maintained by maintaining the realistic perception of reality and avoiding negative outcomes. Statements like, "I am going to maintain my manner of speech and communication possibilities" or "I am a fighter and I will fight the progression of this disease" are both reassuring and hopeful if they are also maintained in a strong reality base. If these statements are not maintained in the base of reality, they can become self-defeating and counterproductive.

8. "IF . . . THEN" CONDITIONAL EVENTS

Hope is sometimes dependent on certain events which may or may not occur. It is important that ALS patients live in the present moment but also be sensitive to hopeful expectations that may occur in the future. ALS patients at times need to say "If and Then" statements and these can be very useful in maintaining future hope. For example, "With this new medical therapy, I am going to wait till the summer vacation is over. If my speech remains the same by the end of summer, then I will return to teaching." Here, returning to teaching is contingent upon the event of speech status at the end of summer.

9. SPECULATIVE COERCION OF REALITY

Hope is maintained by maintaining a realistic perspective, and fantasizing about possible positive outcome. ALS patients are often times quite diligent in maintaining serveillances about new ALS treatments. They may hear about new and innovative treatment modalities through the news service, friends or relatives. ALS patients are frequently compelled to try these new and innovative treatments because of the unavailability of successful treatments at the present moment. This aspect of hope can be utilized constructively if one takes time to clarify the information obtained, and consults with one's personal physician in order to assess its scientific rationale.

10. FUTURE POSSIBILITIES
(SOMEDAY, SOMETHING)

The possibility of a cure is expressed by maintaining hope in future possibilities, such as "Maybe someday, something," "Who knows maybe a cure for ALS will be found." Enhancing one's knowledge about advances in health care in general and about experimental research projects such as the clinical trials including somatren, cyclosporine, TRH, total lymphoid irradiation and branched-chain aminoacids can help to maintain hope. Remaining in close contact with one's physician, keeping periodic follow-up visits at the local ALS clinic and receiving periodic reports from MDA may be positive ways of focusing scientific studies and remaining current with future developments.

11. TRUISM

Uncontestable positive generalities that can apply to a general ALS population can be used to support and maintain hope in ALS patients. For example, "It is possible to live a productive and happy life with ALS if one maintains a strong sense of oneself," or "All that I have to do is to live one day at a time, follow the medical regimen prescribed for me, and to give my best every day." These are very simple positive generalities that can be both comforting and inspiring to ALS patients.

12. HOPE COMMENDATION

ALS patients can be supported by having their hope expectations affirmed. It is important for family, friends and caregivers to listen carefully to the patient's expression of hope. A statement such as, "I get along better with my family when I have a more positive attitude," reveals what the person is hoping for. Listening for these "hope expectations" enables the interpersonal supportive environment to offer various means and methods that may assist the patient in having one's hopes realized. For example, to address the preceding statement, exploring various means of stress management, such as meditation and imagery, may help the patient to maintain a positive attitude. Asking a question such as, "What do you hope for at this time?'' or "What are your expectations?'' may be effective ways to elicit the ALS patient's object of hope. Additionally, it is essential that ALS patients reveal to family, friends and caregivers their hopeful expectations. Helping the ALS patient realize personal hopes and dreams may be an extremely intimate way of conveying love and care to the patient.

13. TESTIMONIAL

The achievements of other ALS patients can also offer support of one's hope. Some ALS patients have been leading productive and happy lives for many years. English physicist Stephen Hawking is a good example. Stephen Hawking contracted ALS when he was pursuing his post graduate work at Cambridge. When he learned that he had ALS and was told it would only get worse, and there was no cure, Hawking was devastated. He felt that there didn't seem to be much point in completing his Ph.D. However, the progression of Hawking's ALS slowed considerably when he found that he had something to live for. With respect to Dr. Hawking, the turning point arrived when he became engaged to his fiancee. Dr. Hawking assumed that if he was to get married, he had to get a job, therefore, he had to finish his Ph.D. That desire motivated him to work very hard for the first time, and at the same time, he was quite surprised to find that he even liked the hard work. After more than 20 years of having ALS, Dr. Hawking is confined to a wheelchair and has a tracheostomy. He is able to communicate through the use of an agonizingly slow computer and depends totally on others for his personal care, and indeed, his very survival. Dr. Hawking is a virtual prisoner in his own body. Nevertheless, he is married, father of two children, wrote a bestseller, and is regarded as one of the leading authorities in the field of physics.

14. THE UNPROMISING FUTURE

The last aspect of hope involves achieving a hopeful attitude by intentionally keeping the future undifferentiated. It is important to keep the future dedifferentiated because of its extremely threatening nature. This is simply an attitude of taking one day at a time. Many ALS patients utilize this method of living for the present in order to maintain a hope in overcoming the formidable future reality. Giving one's best effort, at each moment of the day, is one way of maintaining a hopeful attitude.

These various aspects and methods of instilling hope can be applied in various combinations, with differing emphasis, for each person affected with ALS. Individual differences in hoping styles are to be expected because each hoping style is a unique reflection of the patient's individual personality and differences arising from the patient's immediate environment.

Reality Surveillance

To return to Wright's paradigm, which includes the four cognitive and affective tasks that are present in the hoping process, hopeful expectations have a better opportunity of being actualized for the patient when reality is continually surveyed and assessed. When caregivers, family or friends of ALS patients apply these various hoping styles and methods, it is important to recognize that the patient will often experience different emotions as they progress through the hoping process. The feeling of hope in an individual is comprised of both cognitive process and emotion. During the reality surveillance and assessment, caregivers may often hear expressions that reflect feelings such as fluctuations in attitude, sadness, grief, or mourning of lost skills and abilities expressed by the patient. These expressions of emotions are necessary and extremely important, and serve as products and motivators of hope. These expressions of emotion are also ways that patients establish their own feelings of equilibrium in their own attempts to cognitively evaluate reality.

Encouragement

Feelings of reassurance and encouragement come to patients when they find some base upon which to rest their hope. Encouragement can be provided in the methods outlined above by the patient's interpersonal support network of family, friends and caregivers.

Worrying

ALS patients feel anxious or worried when they are in doubt about whether their hopes can be actualized. While worrying is an uncomfortable feeling, it also has a beneficial side, because it can serve as a motivating factor in enabling the patient to consider various alternative options and treatment modalities that normally may not be utilized.

Mourning

When ALS patients realize that certain hopeful expectations must be discarded or modified, they will often feel sad. They will need to mourn and grieve over the hopeful expectations that have had to be given up. On the other hand, the period of mourning can also be advantageous to the patient because it can provide a time for self-reflection and evaluation. A different perspective and a modification of personal and treatment goals can emerge from this period of self-reflection and evaluation. The patients' sense of their old and familiar self, and hopes, based on their old physical self, can give way to a newly formed realization of their emotional and spiritual self. If the patient can see through the physical walls imposed by ALS which are manifested during this period of mourning, the patient does evolve and emerge with a stronger and happier sense of identity.

SUMMARY

Wright's framework can be extremely useful in assessing ALS patients' cognitive and emotional progression through the course of their disease. As ALS patients progress through their disease, it has been found that cognitive and affective feelings of hope can be extremely useful in maintaining positive medical management, and more importantly, can serve as a way of enhancing and maintaining the patient's positive attitude toward life. These goals may be effectively realized when the patient's interpersonal support network of family, friends and caregivers collaborate and support hopeful expectations for the patient. A number of practical aspects were presented as possible methods that can be utilized by the patients' support network in restoring hope in the patients' attitude toward their disease, ALS, and indeed, life itself.

REFERENCES

Lange, S. P. 1978. "Hope." In C. E. Carlson and B. Blackwell, eds. *Behavioral Concepts and Nursing Intervention*. New York: J.B. Lippincott Co., pp. 171-190.
Wright, B. A. and F. C. Shontz. 1968. "Process and Tasks in Hoping." *Rehabilitation Literature* 29(11): 322-331.

T - #0184 - 101024 - C0 - 229/152/14 [16] - CB - 9781560240778 - Gloss Lamination